NATIONAL HIV/AIDS STRATEGY FOR THE UNITED STATES

JULY 2010

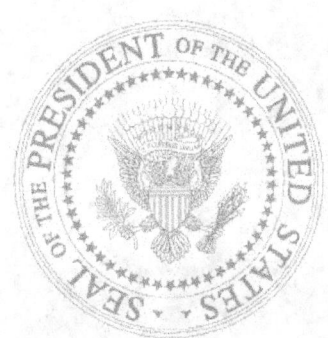

July 13, 2010

Thirty years ago, the first cases of human immunodeficiency virus (HIV) garnered the world's attention. Since then, over 575,000 Americans have lost their lives to AIDS and more than 56,000 people in the United States become infected with HIV each year. Currently, there are more than 1.1 million Americans living with HIV. Moreover, almost half of all Americans know someone living with HIV.

Our country is at a crossroads. Right now, we are experiencing a domestic epidemic that demands a renewed commitment, increased public attention, and leadership. Early in my Administration, I tasked the Office of National AIDS Policy with developing a *National HIV/AIDS Strategy* with three primary goals: 1) reducing the number of people who become infected with HIV; 2) increasing access to care and improving health outcomes for people living with HIV; and, 3) reducing HIV-related health disparities. To accomplish these goals, we must undertake a more coordinated national response to the epidemic. The Federal government can't do this alone, nor should it. Success will require the commitment of governments at all levels, businesses, faith communities, philanthropy, the scientific and medical communities, educational institutions, people living with HIV, and others.

Countless Americans have devoted their lives to fighting the HIV epidemic and thanks to their tireless work we've made real inroads. People living with HIV have transformed how we engage community members in setting policy, conducting research, and providing services. Researchers have produced a wealth of information about the disease, including a number of critical tools and interventions to diagnose, prevent, and treat HIV. Successful prevention efforts have averted more than 350,000 new infections in the United States. And health care and other services providers have taught us how to provide quality services in diverse settings and develop medical homes for people with HIV. This moment represents an opportunity for the Nation. Now is the time to build on and refocus our existing efforts to deliver better results for the American people.

I look forward to working with Congress, State, tribal, and local governments, and other stakeholders to support the implementation of a Strategy that is innovative, grounded in the best science, focuses on the areas of greatest need, and that provides a clear direction for moving forward together.

Vision for the National HIV/AIDS Strategy

"The United States will become a place where new HIV infections are rare and when they do occur, every person, regardless of age, gender, race/ethnicity, sexual orientation, gender identity or socio-economic circumstance, will have unfettered access to high quality, life-extending care, free from stigma and discrimination"

Executive Summary

When one of our fellow citizens becomes infected with the human immunodeficiency virus (HIV) every nine-and-a-half minutes, the epidemic affects all Americans. It has been nearly thirty years since the first cases of HIV garnered the world's attention. Without treatment, the virus slowly debilitates a person's immune system until they succumb to illness. The epidemic has claimed the lives of nearly 600,000 Americans and affects many more.[1] Our Nation is at a crossroads. We have the knowledge and tools needed to slow the spread of HIV infection and improve the health of people living with HIV. Despite this potential, however, the public's sense of urgency associated with combating the epidemic appears to be declining. In 1995, 44 percent of the general public indicated that HIV/AIDS was the most urgent health problem facing the Nation, compared to only 6 percent in March 2009.[2] While HIV transmission rates have been reduced substantially over time and people with HIV are living longer and more productive lives, approximately 56,000 people become infected each year and more Americans are living with HIV than ever before.[3,4] Unless we take bold actions, we face a new era of rising infections, greater challenges in serving people living with HIV, and higher health care costs.[5]

President Obama committed to developing a *National HIV/AIDS Strategy* with three primary goals: 1) reducing the number of people who become infected with HIV, 2) increasing access to care and optimizing health outcomes for people living with HIV, and 3) reducing HIV-related health disparities. To accomplish these goals, we must undertake a more coordinated national response to the HIV epidemic. The Strategy is intended to be a concise plan that will identify a set of priorities and strategic action steps tied to measurable outcomes. Accompanying the Strategy is a Federal Implementation Plan that outlines the specific steps to be taken by various Federal agencies to support the high-level priorities outlined in the Strategy. This is an ambitious plan that will challenge us to meet all of the goals that we set. The job, however, does not fall to the Federal Government alone, nor should it. Success will require the commitment of all parts of society, including State, tribal and local governments, businesses, faith communities, philanthropy, the scientific and medical communities, educational institutions, people living with HIV, and others. The vision for the *National HIV/AIDS Strategy* is simple:

> *The United States will become a place where new HIV infections are rare and when they do occur, every person, regardless of age, gender, race/ethnicity, sexual orientation, gender identity or socio-economic circumstance, will have unfettered access to high quality, life-extending care, free from stigma and discrimination.*

---

1. CDC. *HIV/AIDS Surveillance Report*. 2007; 19: 7. Available at
http://www.cdc.gov/hiv/topics/surveillance/resources/reports/2007report/pdf/2007SurveillanceReport.pdf
2. Kaiser Family Foundation. *2009 Survey of Americans on HIV/AIDS: Summary of Findings on the Domestic Epidemic*. April 2009.
3. CDC. *Estimates of new HIV infections in the United States*. August 2008. Available at
http://www.kff.org/kaiserpolls/upload/7889.pdf
4. CDC. *HIV Prevalence Estimates—United States*, 2006. *MMWR* 2008;57(39):1073-76.
5. If the HIV transmission rate remained constant at 5.0 persons infected each year per 100 people living with HIV, within a decade, the number of new infections would increase to more than 75,000 per year and the number of people living with HIV would grow to more than 1,500,000 (*JAIDS*, in press).

Reducing New HIV Infections

More must be done to ensure that new prevention methods are identified and that prevention resources are more strategically concentrated in specific communities at high risk for HIV infection. Almost half of all Americans know someone living with HIV (43 percent in 2009).[6] Our national commitment to ending the HIV epidemic, however, cannot be tied only to our own perception of how closely HIV affects us personally. Just as we mobilize the country to support cancer prevention and research whether or not we believe that we are at high risk of cancer, or just as we support investments in public education whether or not we have children, success at fighting HIV calls on all Americans to help us sustain a long-term effort against HIV. While anyone can become infected with HIV, some Americans are at greater risk than others. This includes gay and bisexual men of all races and ethnicities, Black men and women, Latinos and Latinas, people struggling with addiction, including injection drug users, and people in geographic hot spots, including the United States South and Northeast, as well as Puerto Rico and the U.S. Virgin Islands. By focusing our efforts in communities where HIV is concentrated, we can have the biggest impact in lowering all communities' collective risk of acquiring HIV.

We must also move away from thinking that one approach to HIV prevention will work, whether it is condoms, pills, or information. Instead, we need to develop, evaluate, and implement effective prevention strategies and combinations of approaches including efforts such as expanded HIV testing (since people who know their status are less likely to transmit HIV), education and support to encourage people to reduce risky behaviors, the strategic use of medications and biomedical interventions (which have allowed us, for example, to nearly eliminate HIV transmission to newborns), the development of vaccines and microbicides, and the expansion of evidence-based mental health and substance abuse prevention and treatment programs. It is essential that all Americans have access to a shared base of factual information about HIV. The Strategy also provides an opportunity for working together to advance a public health approach to sexual health that includes HIV prevention as one component. To successfully reduce the number of new HIV infections, there must be a concerted effort by the public and private sectors, including government at all levels, individuals, and communities, to:

- Intensify HIV prevention efforts in communities where HIV is most heavily concentrated.

- Expand targeted efforts to prevent HIV infection using a combination of effective, evidence-based approaches.

- Educate all Americans about the threat of HIV and how to prevent it.

Increasing Access to Care and Improving Health Outcomes for People Living with HIV

As a result of our ongoing investments in research and years of clinical experience, people living with HIV can enjoy long and healthy lives. To make this a reality for everyone, it is important to get people with HIV into care early after infection to protect their health and reduce their potential of transmitting the virus to others. For these reasons, it is important that all people living with HIV are well supported in a

---

6. Kaiser Family Foundation. 2009 Survey of Americans on HIV/AIDS: Summary of Findings on the Domestic Epidemic. April 2009. Available at http://www.kff.org/kaiserpolls/upload/7889.pdf

regular system of care. The *Affordable Care Act*, which will greatly expand access to insurance coverage for people living with HIV, will provide a platform for improvements in health care coverage and quality. High risk pools are available immediately. High risk pools will be established in every state to provide coverage to uninsured people with chronic conditions. In 2014, Medicaid will be expanded to all lower income individuals (below 133% of the Federal poverty level, or about $15,000 for a single individual in 2010) under age 65. Uninsured people with incomes up to 400% of the Federal poverty level (about $43,000 for a single individual in 2010) will have access to Federal tax credits and the opportunity to purchase private insurance coverage through competitive insurance exchanges. New consumer protections will better protect people with private insurance coverage by ending discrimination based on health status and pre-existing conditions. Gaps in essential care and services for people living with HIV will continue to need to be addressed along with the unique biological, psychological, and social effects of living with HIV. Therefore, the Ryan White HIV/AIDS Program and other Federal and State HIV-focused programs will continue to be necessary after the law is implemented. Additionally, improving health outcomes requires continued investments in research to develop safer, cheaper, and more effective treatments. Both public and private sector entities must take the following steps to improve service delivery for people living with HIV:

- Establish a seamless system to immediately link people to continuous and coordinated quality care when they are diagnosed with HIV.

- Take deliberate steps to increase the number and diversity of available providers of clinical care and related services for people living with HIV.

- Support people living with HIV with co-occurring health conditions and those who have challenges meeting their basic needs, such as housing.

Reducing HIV-Related Health Disparities

The stigma associated with HIV remains extremely high and fear of discrimination causes some Americans to avoid learning their HIV status, disclosing their status, or accessing medical care.[7] Data indicate that HIV disproportionately affects the most vulnerable in our society—those Americans who have less access to prevention and treatment services and, as a result, often have poorer health outcomes. Further, in some heavily affected communities, HIV may not be viewed as a primary concern, such as in communities experiencing problems with crime, unemployment, lack of housing, and other pressing issues. Therefore, to successfully address HIV, we need more and better community-level approaches that integrate HIV prevention and care with more comprehensive responses to social service needs. Key steps for the public and private sector to take to reduce HIV-related health disparities are:

- Reduce HIV-related mortality in communities at high risk for HIV infection.

- Adopt community-level approaches to reduce HIV infection in high-risk communities.

- Reduce stigma and discrimination against people living with HIV.

---

7. Mahajan AP, Sayles JN, Patel VA, et al. Stigma in the HIV/AIDS epidemic: A review of the literature and recommendations for the way forward. *AIDS* 2008;22(Suppl 2):S67-S69.

Achieving a More Coordinated National Response to the HIV Epidemic in the United States

The Nation can succeed at meeting the President's goals. It will require the Federal Government and State, tribal and local governments, however, to do some things differently. Foremost is the need for an unprecedented commitment to collaboration, efficiency, and innovation. We also must be prepared to adjust course as needed. This Strategy is intended to complement other related efforts across the Administration. For example, the *President's Emergency Plan for AIDS Relief (PEPFAR)* has taught us valuable lessons about fighting HIV and scaling up efforts around the world that can be applied to the domestic epidemic. The *President's National Drug Control Strategy* serves as a blueprint for reducing drug use and its consequences, and the *Federal Strategic Plan to Prevent and End Homelessness* focuses efforts to reduce homelessness and increase housing security. The White House Office of National AIDS Policy (ONAP) will work collaboratively with the Office of National Drug Control Policy and other White House offices, as well as relevant agencies to further the goals of the Strategy. The Strategy is intended to promote greater investment in HIV/AIDS, but this is not a budget document. Nonetheless, it will inform the Federal budget development process within the context of the fiscal goals that the President has articulated. The United States currently provides more than $19 billion in annual funding for domestic HIV prevention, care, and research, and there are constraints on the magnitude of any potential new investments in the Federal budget. The Strategy should be used to refocus our existing efforts and deliver better results to the American people within current funding levels, as well as to highlight the need for additional investments. Our national progress will require sustaining broader public commitment to HIV, and this calls for more regular communications to ensure transparency about whether we are meeting national goals. Key steps are to:

- Increase the coordination of HIV programs across the Federal government and between federal agencies and state, territorial, tribal, and local governments.

- Develop improved mechanisms to monitor and report on progress toward achieving national goals.

This Strategy provides a basic framework for moving forward. With government at all levels doing its part, a committed private sector, and leadership from people living with HIV and affected communities, the United States can dramatically reduce HIV transmission and better support people living with HIV and their families.

Introduction

It has been nearly thirty years since the first cases of human immunodeficiency virus (HIV) garnered the world's attention. Without treatment, the virus slowly debilitates a person's immune system until they succumb to illness. The epidemic has claimed the lives of nearly 600,000 Americans and affects many more.[8] Our Nation is at a crossroads: the urgency associated with combating the epidemic appears to be declining as people with HIV live longer and more productive lives. In 1995, 44 percent of the general public indicated that HIV/AIDS was the most urgent health problem facing the Nation, compared to only six percent in March 2009.[9] Approximately 56,000 people become infected each year, and more than 1.1 million Americans are living with HIV.[10,11] Unless we take bold actions, however, we anticipate a new era of rising infections and even greater challenges in serving people living with HIV.[12]

President Obama committed to developing a *National HIV/AIDS Strategy* with three primary goals:

- Reducing the number of people who become infected with HIV;

- Increasing access to care and optimizing health outcomes for people living with HIV; and,

- Reducing HIV-related health disparities.

To accomplish these goals, we must achieve a more coordinated national response to the HIV epidemic.

Where Things Stand: HIV in the United States

Although the United States has accomplished many successes in fighting HIV, much more needs to be done to curb the epidemic. Research has produced a wealth of information about HIV disease, including a number of critical tools and interventions to diagnose, prevent, and treat HIV infection. HIV transmission rates have been dramatically reduced in the United States and people with HIV are living healthier and more productive lives than ever before. Nevertheless, much more needs to be done. With more than one million Americans living with HIV, there are more people in need of testing, prevention, and treatment services than at any point in history, and ongoing research efforts are needed to find a cure for HIV/AIDS and continue to develop improved prevention tools and effective treatments. The Strategy cannot succeed without continued and sustained progress in biomedical and behavioral research.

The challenges we face are sobering:

- Approximately one in five people living with HIV are unaware of their status, placing them at greater risk for spreading the virus to others.[13]

---

8. CDC. *HIV/AIDS Surveillance Report.* 2007; 19: 7. Available at
http://www.cdc.gov/hiv/topics/surveillance/resources/reports/2007report/pdf/2007SurveillanceReport.pdf
9. Kaiser Family Foundation. *2009 Survey of Americans on HIV/AIDS: Summary of Findings on the Domestic Epidemic.* April 2009.
Available at http://www.kff.org/kaiserpolls/upload/7889.pdf
10. Hall HI, Song R, Rhodes P, et al. Estimation of HIV incidence in the United States. *JAMA* 2008;300(5):520-529.
11. CDC. *HIV Prevalence Estimates—United States, 2006. MMWR* 2008;57(39):1073-76.
12. If the HIV transmission rate remained constant at 5.0 persons infected each year per 100 people living with HIV, within a decade, the number of new infections would increase to more than 75,000 per year, and the number of people living with HIV would grow to more than 1,500,000 (JAIDS, in press).
13. CDC. *Estimates of new HIV infections in the United States.* August 2008. Available at
www.cdc.gov/hiv/topics/surveillance/resources/factsheets/pdf/incidence.pdf

- Roughly three-fourths of HIV/AIDS cases in the United States are among men, the majority of whom are gay and bisexual men.[14,15]

- One-fourth of Americans living with HIV are women, and the disease disproportionately impacts women of color. The HIV diagnosis rate for Black women is more than 19 times the rate for White women.[16,17]

- Racial and ethnic minorities are disproportionately represented in the HIV epidemic and die sooner than Whites. [18,19]

- The South and Northeast, along with Puerto Rico and the U.S. Virgin Islands, are disproportionately impacted by HIV.[20]

- One quarter of new HIV infections occur among adolescents and young adults (ages 13 to 29).[21]

- Twenty-four percent of people living with HIV are 50 or older, and 15 percent of new HIV/AIDS cases occur among people in this age group.[22]

Development of the National HIV/AIDS Strategy

Since taking office, the Obama Administration has worked to engage the public to evaluate what we are doing right and identify new approaches that will strengthen our response to the domestic epidemic. The White House Office of National AIDS Policy (ONAP), a component of the Domestic Policy Council, has been tasked with leading the effort to develop a national strategy. Throughout the process, ONAP has taken steps to engage as many Americans as possible to hear their ideas for making progress in the fight against HIV. ONAP's outreach included hosting 14 HIV/AIDS Community Discussions with thousands of people across the United States, reviewing suggestions from the public via the White House website, conducting a series of expert meetings on several HIV-specific topics, and working with Federal and community partners who organized their own meetings to support the development of a national strategy. A report summarizing public recommendations for the strategy, entitled *Community Ideas for Improving the Response to the Domestic HIV Epidemic*, was published in April 2010.[23]

---

14. CDC. *HIV/AIDS Surveillance Report.* 2007; 19: 7. Available at
http://www.cdc.gov/hiv/topics/surveillance/resources/reports/2007report/pdf/2007SurveillanceReport.pdf
15. Throughout this document we use the terms "gay and bisexual men" and "gay men" interchangeably, and we intend these terms to be inclusive of all men who have sex with men (MSM), even those who do not identify as gay or bisexual.
16. Throughout this document we use the terms "Black" and "African American" interchangeably, and we intend these terms to be inclusive of all individuals from the African Diaspora who identify as Black and/or African American.
17. CDC. HIV and AIDS in the United States: A Picture of Today's Epidemic. 2007. Available at
http://www.cdc.gov/hiv/topics/surveillance/united_states.htm
18. CDC. *HIV/AIDS Surveillance Report.* 2007; 19: 7. Available at
http://www.cdc.gov/hiv/topics/surveillance/resources/reports/2007report/pdf/2007SurveillanceReport.pdf
19. Losina E, Schackman BR, Sadownik SN, et al. Racial and Sex Disparities in Life Expectancy Losses among HIV-Infected Persons in the United States. *Clin Infect Dis* 2009;49(10):1570-8.
20. CDC. *HIV/AIDS Surveillance Report.* 2007; 19: 7. Available at
http://www.cdc.gov/hiv/topics/surveillance/resources/reports/2007report/pdf/2007SurveillanceReport.pdf
21. CDC. *Estimates of new HIV infections in the United States.* August 2008. Available at
www.cdc.gov/hiv/topics/surveillance/resources/factsheets/pdf/incidence.pdf
22. CDC. HIV and AIDS among persons aged 50 and over. 2008. Available at
www.cdc.gov/hiv/topics/over50/resources/factsheets/pdf/over50.pdf. Accessed February 18, 2010.
23. See www.WhiteHouse.gov/ONAP.

To develop the Strategy, ONAP convened a panel of Federal officials from across government to assist in reviewing the public recommendations, assessing the scientific evidence for or against various recommendations, and making their own recommendations for the Strategy. ONAP also has contracted with the Institute of Medicine to examine several key policy issues.

This document provides a roadmap to move the Nation forward in responding to the domestic HIV epidemic. It is not intended to be a comprehensive list of all activities needed to address HIV/AIDS in the United States, but is intended to be a concise plan that identifies a set of priorities and strategic action steps tied to measurable outcomes. The *National HIV/AIDS Strategy* outlines top-line priorities. Additional details on the specific actions that the Federal Government will take to implement its part of the Strategy are included in a *Federal Implementation Plan*. This is an ambitious plan that will challenge us to meet all of the goals that we set. Both the *National HIV/AIDS Strategy* and the *Federal Implementation Plan* may be accessed at www.WhiteHouse.gov/ONAP.

The job of implementing the *National HIV/AIDS Strategy*, however, does not fall to the Federal Government alone, nor should it. Success will require the commitment of all parts of society, including State, tribal and local governments, businesses, faith communities, philanthropy, the scientific and medical communities, educational institutions, people living with HIV, and others.

Reducing New HIV Infections

The Opportunity

Within a few short years in the 1980s, HIV went from an unknown condition to an epidemic that was infecting more than 130,000 people annually.[24] The United States succeeded in mounting a response that involved affected communities, businesses, the public sector, foundations, pharmaceutical companies, scientific, medical, and public health professionals, faith communities, and others. These collective efforts were important for helping to reduce HIV infection rates. By 2000, the number of Americans becoming infected each year had fallen to an estimated 56,300.[25] Activities that contributed to our success in reducing HIV infections include:

- **HIV testing:** HIV testing has enabled individuals with HIV to become aware of their health status and to take appropriate precautions to preserve their health. Moreover, studies show that individuals diagnosed with HIV take steps to reduce the likelihood of transmitting HIV to others.

- **Effective screening of the blood supply:** Early in the epidemic, people contracted HIV through blood transfusions, but because of government research and the implementation of effective blood screening procedures, HIV transmission through blood transfusion is very rare.[26,27]

- **Screening and treating expectant mothers during pregnancy:** Government-sponsored research in the 1990s demonstrated that taking antiretroviral medication prevents HIV transmission from mother to child during pregnancy and delivery. Cases declined from an estimated 1,650 a year in 1991 to fewer than 200 per year by 2004.[28]

24. Hall HI, Song R, Rhodes P, et al. Estimation of HIV incidence in the United States. *JAMA* 2008;300(5):520-529.
25. Hall HI, Song R, Rhodes P, et al. Estimation of HIV incidence in the United States. *JAMA* 2008;300(5):520-529.
26. CDC. HIV and AIDS-United States, 1981-2000. *MMWR* 2001 50(21);430-4.
27. Phelps R, Robbins K, Liberti T, et al. Window-period human immunodeficiency virus transmission to two recipients by an adolescent blood donor. *Transfusion.* 2004;44:929-933.
28. CDC. HIV/AIDS Fact Sheet: Pregnancy and Childbirth. 2007. Available at http://www.cdc.gov/hiv/topics/perinatal/overview_partner.htm

- **Minimizing infections from injection drug use:** Comprehensive, evidence-based drug prevention and treatment strategies have contributed to reducing HIV infections. In 1993, injection drug users comprised 31 percent of AIDS cases nationally compared to 17 percent by 2007.[29] Studies show that comprehensive prevention and drug treatment programs, including needle exchange, have dramatically cut the number of new HIV infections among people who inject drugs by 80 percent since the mid-1990s.[30,31,32]

- **Advances in HIV therapies:** HIV medications can extend the length and quality of life for infected individuals, and lower the amount of the virus circulating in a person's body, thereby reducing their risk of transmitting HIV to others.[33]

Because of these and other prevention efforts, the annual number of new infections has not risen despite a growing number of people living with HIV, and thus, a larger pool of people capable of transmitting HIV to others (Figure 1). Unless we mount more intensive prevention efforts and keep innovating to develop more and better prevention methods, the number of new HIV infections will likely rise.[34]

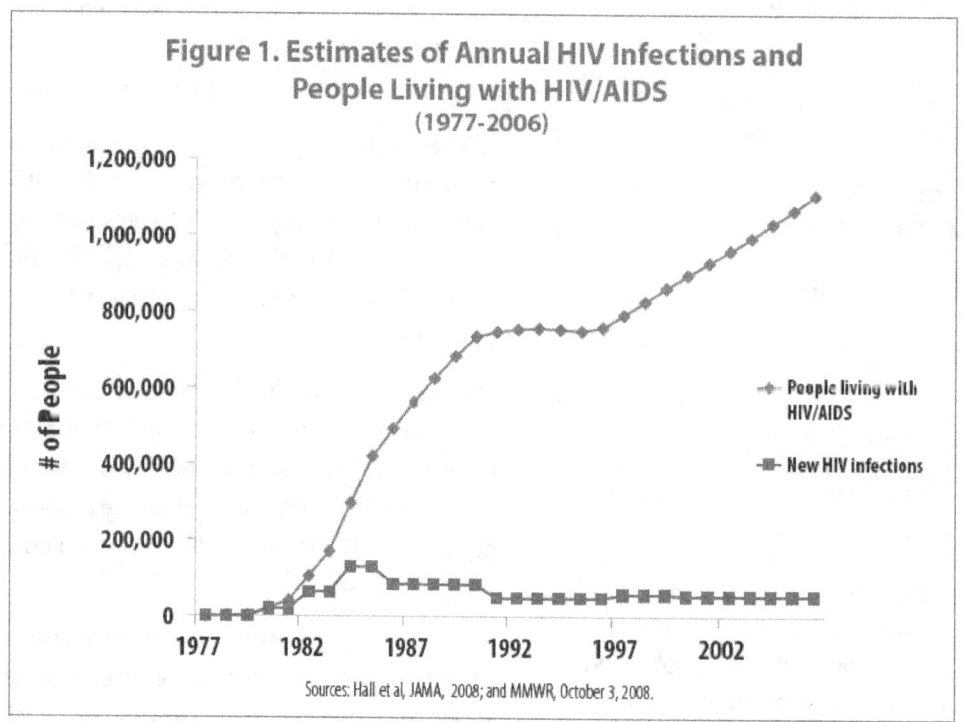

Figure 1. Estimates of Annual HIV Infections and People Living with HIV/AIDS (1977-2006)

Sources: Hall et al, JAMA, 2008; and MMWR, October 3, 2008.

The following are challenges that must be overcome:

29. CDC. HIV/AIDS Surveillance in Injection Drug Users (through 2007). Available at http://www.cdc.gov/hiv/idu/resources/slides/index.htm

30. Des Jarlais DC, Perlis T, Kamyar A, et al. HIV Incidence Among Injection Drug Users in New York City, 1990 to 2002: Use of Serologic Test Algorithm to Assess Expansion of HIV Prevention Services. *Am J Public Health*. 2005;95:1439-1444.

31. Strathdee SA, Patrick DM, Currie SL, et al. Needle exchange is not enough: lessons from the Vancouver injecting drug use study. *AIDS*. 1997;11:F59-65

32. CDC. HIV infection among injection-drug users—34 States, 2004-2007. *MMWR*. 2009;58:1291-1295.

33. Donnell D, Baeten JM, Kiarie J, et al. Heterosexual HIV-1 transmission after initiation of antiretroviral therapy: a prospective cohort analysis. *Lancet*. 2010.

34. If the HIV transmission rate remained constant at 5.0 persons infected each year per 100 people living with HIV, within a decade, the number of new infections would increase to more than 75,000 per year and the number of people living with HIV would grow to more than 1,500,000 (*JAIDS*, in press).

- **Too many people living with HIV are unaware of their status:** An estimated 21 percent of people with HIV in the United States do not know their status.[35] Studies show that people who do not know that they are HIV-positive are more likely to engage in risk behaviors associated with HIV transmission.[36] Some of these individuals are already accessing health care services, but opportunities to diagnose them are being missed.[37]

- **Access to HIV prevention is too limited:** HIV prevention services have never been sufficient to reach all people at risk for HIV. Since Federal resources are limited and many States have reduced HIV prevention budgets in response to the economic downturn, we need to do a better job of evaluating and allocating existing resources based on their demonstrated health impact.

- **Insufficient access to care:** HIV medications not only improve the health of the individual, they also reduce their infectiousness, reducing their risk of transmitting HIV to others. An estimated one-third of people living with HIV in the United States are not in care.[38] Large numbers of uninsured and underinsured people with HIV mean that not everyone has sufficient access to HIV therapy.

- **Diminished public attention:** Media and public attention to the HIV epidemic has waned. The Kaiser Family Foundation found that in 2009, only 45 percent of respondents in a poll of the general public said that they had heard "some" or "a lot" about the problems of AIDS in the United States in the last year, compared to 70 percent of respondents in 2004.[39] Because HIV is treatable, many people now think that it is no longer a public health emergency.

HIV infection is preventable. Allowing the number of new infections to rise or remain the same imposes costs on the country because the lifetime cost of treating HIV is estimated to be approximately $355,000 per person.[40] If we do not substantially reduce HIV incidence in the United States, the numbers of people living with HIV and the cost of their care will continue to grow. We need to get better results from existing resources, and promote new investments from Federal, State, tribal, and local governments, as well as philanthropy, businesses, and community resources to achieve the goals that we set.

Steps To Be Taken

There are three critical steps that we must take to reduce HIV infections:

1. Intensify HIV prevention efforts in communities where HIV is most heavily concentrated.

2. Expand targeted efforts to prevent HIV infection using a combination of effective, evidence-based approaches.

3. Educate all Americans about the threat of HIV and how to prevent it.

---

35. CDC. HIV prevalence estimates—United States, 2006. *MMWR*. 2008; 57: 1073-1076.

36. Marks G, Crepaz N, Janssen RS. Estimating sexual transmission of HIV from persons aware and unaware that they are infected with the virus in the USA. AIDS 2006; 26;10:1447-50.

37. Jenkins TC, Gardener EM, Thrun MW, et al., Risk-Based Human Immunodeficiency Virus (HIV) Testing Fails to Detect the Majority of HIV-Infected Persons in Medical Care Settings. *Sex Transm Dis*. 2006; 33:329-333.

38. HRSA. HIV/AIDS Bureau. Outreach: Engaging People in HIV Care. August 2006. Available at http://hab.hrsa.gov/tools/HIVoutreach

39. Kaiser Family Foundation. *2009 Survey of Americans on HIV/AIDS: Summary of Findings on the Domestic Epidemic*. April 2009. Available at http://www.kff.org/kaiserpolls/upload/7889.pdf

40. Schackman BR, Gebo KA, Walensky RP, et al. The lifetime cost of current human immunodeficiency virus care in the United States. *Med Care* 2006;44(11):990-97.

Anticipated Results

By working together, we hope to meet the following benchmarks by 2015:[41]

- Lower the annual number of new infections by 25 percent (from 56,300 to 42,225);

- Reduce the HIV transmission rate, which is a measure of annual transmissions in relation to the number of people living with HIV, by 30 percent (from 5 persons infected each year per 100 people with HIV to 3.5 persons infected each year per 100 people with HIV); and,

- Increase from 79 percent to 90 percent the percentage of people living with HIV who know their serostatus (from 948,000 to 1,080,000 people).

Recommended Actions

Step 1: Intensify HIV prevention efforts in the communities where HIV is most heavily concentrated.
In the beginning of the HIV epidemic, there was widespread fear that the epidemic would spread to the general population. The public heard about growing infection rates and that HIV had spread to all parts of the country. While this is true, nearly three decades later, the U.S. epidemic has not run the course that was previously feared. In contrast to HIV epidemics in sub-Saharan Africa and parts of Asia where nearly all sexually active adults are at high risk of becoming infected, HIV cases in the United States are concentrated in specific locations and populations.[42] More must be done to ensure that prevention resources are more strategically concentrated in specific communities at high risk for HIV infection.

Almost half of all Americans know someone living with HIV (43 percent in 2009), but our national commitment to ending the HIV epidemic cannot be tied only to perceptions of how closely HIV affects us personally.[43] All Americans have a stake in preventing HIV transmission and need to remain invested in sustaining our collective efforts to reduce HIV transmission. By intensifying our efforts in communities where HIV is concentrated, however, we can have the biggest impact that will lower all communities' collective risk of acquiring HIV infection. Just as we mobilize the country to support cancer prevention and research whether or not we believe that we are at high risk of cancer and we support public education whether or not we have children, fighting HIV requires widespread public support to sustain a long-term effort. **Not every person or group has an equal chance of becoming infected with HIV.** Yet, for many years, too much of our Nation's response has been conducted as though everyone is equally at risk for HIV infection.

Stopping HIV transmission requires that we focus more intently on the groups and communities where the most cases of new infections are occurring (Figure 2). These numbers alone, however, do not give a complete picture of which populations are at greatest relative risk. Figure 3 shows how the number of new infections in the high-risk groups listed in Figure 2 compares to the total size of each population. Estimating the size of some high-risk populations is challenging and group sizes may be imprecise. Nevertheless, it is clear that some communities are heavily disproportionately impacted compared to others. While we must focus most heavily on those groups with the largest numbers of new infections

---

41. For more information about how these and other targets in the *National HIV/AIDS Strategy* were derived, see the National HIV/AIDS Strategy: Federal Implementation Plan at www.WhiteHouse.gov/ONAP. All numbers are based on current estimates.

42. El-Sadr W, Mayer KH, Hodder SL. AIDS in America—Forgotten but not Gone. *New Engl J Med.* 2010.

43. Kaiser Family Foundation. *2009 Survey of Americans on HIV/AIDS: Summary of Findings on the Domestic Epidemic.* April 2009. Available at http://www.kff.org/kaiserpolls/upload/7889.pdf

(Figure 2), the estimated relative risk of infection helps us to better understand disparities among these populations and how to prioritize efforts between and within groups (Figure 3). Further, some groups may be at very high risk of infection in relation to their group size, but they contribute relatively few cases to national totals of new infections. For example, Figure 3 shows that Black male and female injection drug users are at the greatest risk for new HIV infection relative to their population size, but, as indicated in Figure 2, they represent a small fraction of new infections each year among the highest risk groups. Some other groups not shown here may be at high risk of infection in relation to their population size, but they contribute fewer cases to national totals of new infections (e.g. Latino[44] injection drug users).

---

44. Throughout this document we use the terms "Latino" and "Hispanic" interchangeably. "Hispanic" is used in the Figures to match data sources.

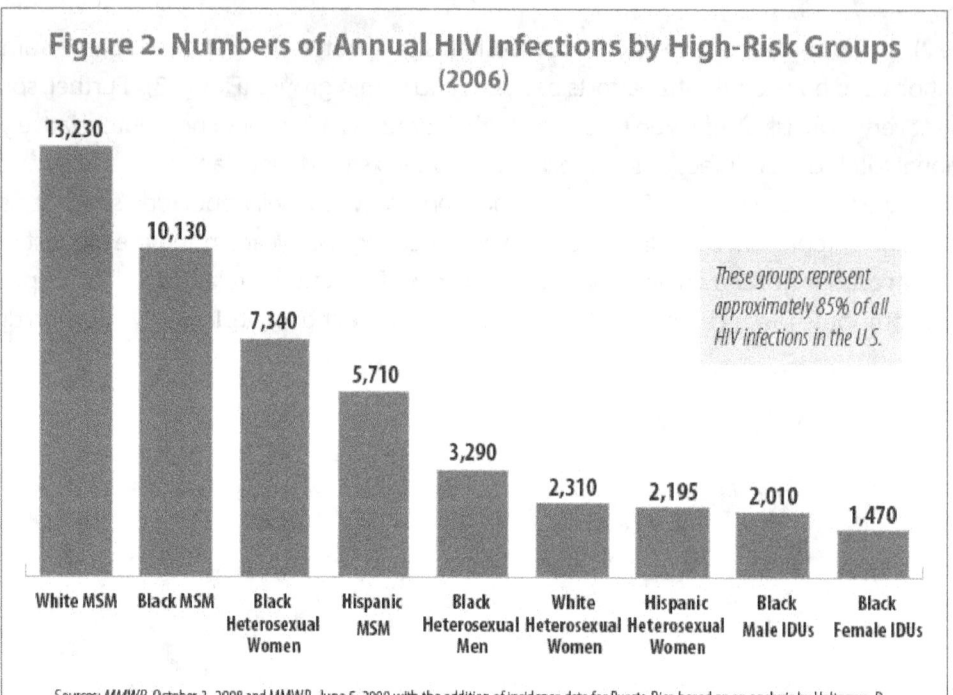

Figure 2. Numbers of Annual HIV Infections by High-Risk Groups
(2006)

These groups represent approximately 85% of all HIV infections in the U.S.

White MSM	13,230
Black MSM	10,130
Black Heterosexual Women	7,340
Hispanic MSM	5,710
Black Heterosexual Men	3,290
White Heterosexual Women	2,310
Hispanic Heterosexual Women	2,195
Black Male IDUs	2,010
Black Female IDUs	1,470

Sources: *MMWR*, October 3, 2008 and MMWR, June 5, 2009 with the addition of incidence data for Puerto Rico based on an analysis by Holtgrave, D., Johns Hopkins Bloomberg School of Public Health. For this analysis, all Puerto Rico cases were classified as Hispanic. Chart based upon CDC, *HIV Prevention in the United States at a Critical Crossroads*, 2009. MSM = men who have sex with men (gay and bisexual men) and IDUs = injection drug users.

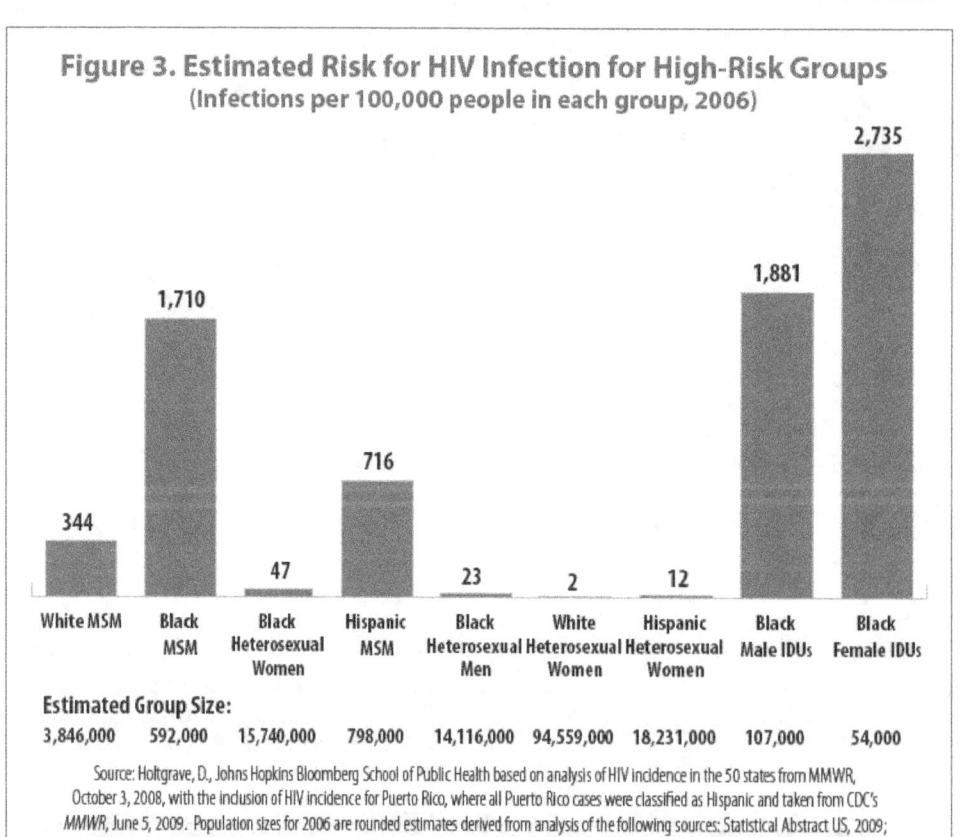

Figure 3. Estimated Risk for HIV Infection for High-Risk Groups
(Infections per 100,000 people in each group, 2006)

White MSM	344
Black MSM	1,710
Black Heterosexual Women	47
Hispanic MSM	716
Black Heterosexual Men	23
White Heterosexual Women	2
Hispanic Heterosexual Women	12
Black Male IDUs	1,881
Black Female IDUs	2,735

Estimated Group Size:

White MSM	Black MSM	Black Heterosexual Women	Hispanic MSM	Black Heterosexual Men	White Heterosexual Women	Hispanic Heterosexual Women	Black Male IDUs	Black Female IDUs
3,846,000	592,000	15,740,000	798,000	14,116,000	94,559,000	18,231,000	107,000	54,000

Source: Holtgrave, D., Johns Hopkins Bloomberg School of Public Health based on analysis of HIV incidence in the 50 states from MMWR, October 3, 2008, with the inclusion of HIV incidence for Puerto Rico, where all Puerto Rico cases were classified as Hispanic and taken from CDC's *MMWR*, June 5, 2009. Population sizes for 2006 are rounded estimates derived from analysis of the following sources: Statistical Abstract US, 2009; CDC estimate of 4% of men are MSM (MSM denotes men who have sex with men); The National Survey on Drug Use and Health Report, October 29, 2009; Brady et al., *Journal of Urban Health* 2008; and Thierry et al., *Emerging Infectious Diseases*, 2004.

At a time of limited resources, we must re-orient our efforts by giving much more attention and resources to the following populations at highest risk of HIV infection:

- **Gay and bisexual men:** According to the Centers for Disease Control and Prevention, gay men comprise approximately 2 percent of the U.S. population, but 53 percent of new infections.[45] Among gay men, White gay men constitute the greatest number of new infections, but Black and Latino gay men are at disproportionate risk for infection;[46]

- **Black men and women:** Black men and women represent only 13 percent of the population, but account for 46% of people living with HIV.[47] Among Blacks, gay and bisexual men are at greatest risk for HIV infection followed by women, and heterosexual men.[48] One study of five major cities found that nearly 50 percent of all Black gay and bisexual men were HIV-positive.[49] Sixty-four percent of all women living with HIV/AIDS are Black.[50]

- **Latinos and Latinas:** According to the CDC, the rate of new AIDS diagnoses among Latino men is three times that of White men, and the rate among Latinas is five times that of White women.[51] Gay and bisexual men represent the greatest proportion of HIV cases among Latinos followed by heterosexual Latinas.[52]

- **Substance abusers:** People who inject drugs are a relatively small share of the U.S. population, but they are disproportionately represented in the HIV epidemic. It is estimated that there are about 1 million injection drug users (IDUs), but injection drug use accounts for approximately 16 percent of new HIV infections in the United States [53,54] Although Figure 2 reflects new HIV cases among injection drug users, use of non-injection drugs such as methamphetamine, amyl

45. CDC Press release. CDC analysis provides new look at disproportionate impact of HIV and syphilis among U.S. gay and bisexual men. March 19, 2010. Available at http://www.cdc.gov/nchhstp/newsroom/msmpressrelease.html This press release includes data from the CDC that is based on the most comprehensive analysis to date of nationally representative surveys. The estimate of 2% is based on a range of 1.4-2.7% in the overall U.S. population age 13 and older who have engaged in same sex behavior in the last five years. (Data source: DW Purcell, C Johnson, A Lansky, et al. Calculating HIV and Syphilis Rates for Risk Groups: Estimating the National Population Size of Men Who Have Sex with Men 2010 National STD Prevention Conference; Atlanta, GA Latebreaker #22896 Presented March 10, 2010).

46. CDC. HIV Prevention in the United States at a Critical Crossroads. 2009. Available at http://www.cdc.gov/hiv/resources/reports/pdf/hiv_prev_us.pdf

47. CDC Fact Sheet. HIV/AIDS among African Americans. August 2009. Available at http://www.cdc.gov/hiv/topics/aa/resources/factsheets/aa.htm

48. CDC. HIV Prevention in the United States at a Critical Crossroads. 2009. Available at http://www.cdc.gov/hiv/resources/reports/pdf/hiv_prev_us.pdf

49. CDC. HIV Prevalence, Unrecognized Infection, and HIV Testing Among Men Who Have Sex with Men - Five U.S. Cities, June 2004-April 2005. *MMWR* Weekly 54(24);597-601.

50. CDC Fact Sheet. *HIV/AIDS Among Women*, August 2008. Available at http://www.cdc.gov/hiv/topics/women/resources/factsheets/pdf/women.pdf

51. CDC Fact Sheet. HIV/AIDS among Hispanics/Latinos. 2009. Available at http://www.cdc.gov/hiv/hispanics/resources/factsheets/hispanic.htm

52. CDC. HIV Prevention in the United States at a Critical Crossroads. 2009. Available at http://www.cdc.gov/hiv/resources/reports/pdf/hiv_prev_us.pdf

53. Brady JE, Friedman SR, Cooper HLF, et al. Risk-based prevalence of infection drug users in the U.S. and in large U.S. metropolitan areas from 1992-2002. *J Urban Health*.2008;85:323-351.

54. Hall HI, Song R, Rhodes P, et al. Estimation of HIV incidence in the United States. *JAMA* 2008;300(5):520-529.

nitrites and other drugs are also associated with sexual transmission of HIV infection and should be targeted with prevention efforts.[55,56,57]

Many individuals in these groups may not engage in greater risk behaviors than others, but they still can be more likely to become infected with HIV. Research has shown that the higher risk for these groups is associated with the sheer number of HIV-positive persons in the communities where they live. As a result, any instance of risk behavior carries a far greater likelihood of infection than other communities with fewer cases of HIV. Thus, unprotected sex even once for individuals in some communities carries a greater risk of HIV infection than for individuals in other communities.[58,59] The Northeast and the South, as well as Puerto Rico and the U.S. Virgin Islands, are more impacted by HIV than other parts of the country. [60,61]

Women and men have different biological, psychological, and cultural factors that increase their vulnerability to infection and disease progression. Additional research is needed into the unique factors that place women at risk for HIV infection. Since most infections among women occur through heterosexual sex, their risk is predicated on the risk behaviors of their male partners. This raises complex policy and research questions, as negotiating safer sexual practices can be especially challenging for women who may be vulnerable to physical violence, or who may be emotionally or economically dependent on men.[62] Given the extreme disparities in infection rates among Black women and Latinas when compared to White women, it is also important to consider the unique factors that place them at higher risk for infection. One such issue, although certainly not the only one, relates to a higher proportion of injection drug use by their male partners than in other communities.[63] Another issue involves trying to assess the effect of incarceration on these communities and the impact it has on HIV transmission. Although the available data suggests that relatively few infections occur in prison settings, there is evidence that some people with HIV who had received medical care while incarcerated have difficulty accessing HIV medications upon release—affecting their health and potentially increasing the likelihood that they will transmit HIV.[64,65,66] High rates of incarceration within certain communities can also be destabilizing. When large numbers of men are incarcerated, the gender imbalance in the communities they leave behind can fuel HIV transmissions by increasing the likelihood that the remaining men will have

55. Strathdee SA, Sherman SG. The role of sexual transmission of HIV infection among injection and non-injection drug users. *J Urban Health*. 2003; 80:iii7-14.

56. Molitor F, Truax SR, Ruiz JD, Sun RK. Association of methamphetamine use during sex with risky sexual behaviors and HIV infection among non-injection drug users. *West J Med*. 1998;168(2):93-97.

57. Buchbinder SP, Vittinghoff E, Heagerty P, et al. Sexual Risk, Nitrite Inhalant Use, and Lack of Circumcision associated with HIV Seroconversion in Men who have Sex with Men in the United States. *J Acquir Immune Def Syn*. 2005;39(1):82-89.

58. Millett GA, Flores SA, Peterson J, Bakeman R. Explaining disparities in HIV infection among Black and White men who have sex with men: A meta-analysis of HIV risk behaviors. *AIDS* 2007;21(15): 2083-2091.

59. Hallfors DD, Iritani BJ, Miller WC, Bauer DJ. Sexual and Drug Behavior Patterns and HIV/STD Racial Disparities: The Need for New Directions. *Am J Public Health*. 2007;97(1):125-132.

60. CDC. HIV/AIDS Surveillance in Urban and Nonurban Areas (through 2007) Slide Set. 2009. Available at http://www.cdc.gov/hiv/topics/surveillance/resources/slides/urban-nonurban/index.htm

61. HHS Fact Sheet: HIV/AIDS in the Caribbean. Available at http://www.kff.org/hivaids/upload/7505-06.pdf

62. Amaro H, Raj A. One the margin: Power and women's HIV risk reduction strategies. Sex Roles. 2000;42:723-749.

63. CDC. HIV/AIDS Surveillance in Injection Drug Users (through 2007) Slide set. Available at http://www.cdc.gov/hiv/idu/resources/slides/index.htm

64. CDC. HIV Transmission among Male Inmates in a State Prison System—Georgia, 1992-2005. 2006. Available at http://www.cdc.gov/mmwr/preview/mmwrhtml/mm5515a1.htm.Accessed June 14, 2010.

65. Federal Bureau Of Prisons. HIV Seroconversion Study. Presented at International Emerging Infectious Diseases Conference. March 19-22, Atlanta, GA. 2006.

66. Baillargeon J, Giordano TP, Rich JD, et al. Accessing antiretroviral therapy following release from prison. *JAMA* 2009;301(8):848-857.

multiple, concurrent relationships with female sex partners. This, in turn, increases the likelihood that a single male would transmit HIV to multiple female partners.[67]

Another challenge for policy makers is how to appropriately respond to HIV in communities that represent a small share of the U.S. population. For example, although Asian Americans and Pacific Islanders (AAPIs) represent approximately one percent of HIV/AIDS cases nationally, the numbers of HIV/AIDS cases may be larger because of underreporting or mistakenly classifying Asian HIV cases under another racial category. [68] In addition, when the size of the population is taken into account, American Indians and Alaska Natives (AI/AN) have ranked third behind Blacks and Latinos in rates of HIV/AIDS diagnoses.[69] Although we must focus our national efforts in those communities with the highest numbers of new infections, targeted surveillance efforts must continue to be supported in localities with concentrations of AAPI and Native American communities.

It is clear that African Americans overall and gay and bisexual men (irrespective of race or ethnicity) continue to bear the brunt of HIV infections in the United States. In recent years, policy makers, community leaders and others have begun to mobilize responses to HIV among African Americans. Black Americans represent 13 percent of the U.S. population, but 46 percent of the estimated 1.1 million people living with HIV in the United States are Black.[70] AIDS cases among African Americans surpassed AIDS cases among Whites in 1994 and have steadily increased.[71] Blacks comprise the greatest proportion of HIV/AIDS cases across many transmission categories, including among women, heterosexual men, injection drug users, and infants. HIV/AIDS case rates among Black women are almost twenty times higher than among White women.[72] What is sometimes less recognized is the extent to which the HIV epidemic among African Americans remains concentrated among Black gay men, who comprise the single largest group of African Americans living with HIV.[73] Fighting HIV among African Americans is not mutually exclusive with fighting HIV among gay and bisexual men. Efforts to reduce HIV among Blacks must confront the epidemic among Black gay and bisexual men as forcefully as existing efforts to confront the epidemic among other groups. These overlapping communities both need intensive efforts to stem HIV infection.

Gay and bisexual men have comprised the largest proportion of the HIV epidemic in the United States since the first cases were reported in the 1980s, and that has not changed. They still comprise the greatest proportion of infections nationally. Although not reflected in Figures 2 or 3 because of small numbers, gay and bisexual men also represent the greatest proportion of HIV cases in the AAPI

67. Adimora AA, Schoenbach VJ, Doherty IA. HIV and African Americans in the Southern United States: Sexual Networks and Social Context. *Sex Transm Dis.* 2006; 33(7):S39-S45.

68. CDC Fact Sheet. HIV/AIDS among Asians and Pacific Islanders. August 2008. Available at http://www.cdc.gov/hiv/resources/factsheets/API.htm

69. CDC Fact Sheet. HIV/AIDS among American Indians and Alaska Natives. August 2008. Available at http://www.cdc.gov/hiv/resources/factsheets/aian.htm

70. CDC Fact Sheet. HIV/AIDS among African-Americans. August 2009. Available at http://www.cdc.gov/hiv/topics/aa/resources/factsheets/aa.htm

71. CDC. HIV/AIDS Surveillance by Race/Ethnicity (through 2007) Slide set. April 2009. Available at http://www.cdc.gov/hiv/topics/surveillance/resources/slides/race-ethnicity/index.htm

72. CDC. *HIV/AIDS Surveillance Report.* 2007; 19:7. Available at http://www.cdc.gov/hiv/topics/surveillance/resources/reports/2007report/pdf/2007SurveillanceReport.pdf

73. CDC. HIV Prevention in the United States at a Critical Crossroads. 2009. Available at http://www.cdc.gov/hiv/resources/reports/pdf/hiv_prev_us.pdf

community and in AI/AN communities.[74,75] Given the starkness and the enduring nature of the disparate impact on gay and bisexual men, it is important to significantly reprioritize resources and attention on this community. **The United States cannot reduce the number of HIV infections nationally without better addressing HIV among gay and bisexual men.** Our national commitment to this population has not always reached a level of HIV prevention funding reflective of their risk.[76] Even though gay and bisexual men comprise only two percent of the U.S. population (4 percent of men):

- Gay and bisexual men of all races are the only group in the United States where the estimated number of new HIV infections is rising annually.[77]

- They are 44 to 86 times more likely to become infected with HIV than other men, and 40 to 77 times more likely to become infected than women.[78]

- Approximately one-half of the 1.1 million persons living with HIV in the United States are gay and bisexual men, and they account for the majority (53 percent) of new HIV infections each year.[79]

- High rates of HIV among gay men are found not only in large urban areas. More than half of all AIDS cases diagnosed in the United States are among gay and bisexual men irrespective of town or city size.[80]

As with gay and bisexual men, transgender individuals are also at high risk for HIV infection. Some studies have found that as many as 30 percent of transgender individuals are HIV-positive.[81] Yet, historically, efforts targeting this specific population have been minimal.

The burden of addressing the HIV epidemic among gay and bisexual men and transgender individuals does not rest with the government alone. Early in the epidemic, the lesbian, gay, bisexual and transgender (LGBT) community developed its own education campaigns and institutions to reduce HIV infection in the wake of inaction by government and other institutions. Continuing these efforts is important to our success. Despite our earlier achievements, CDC reports that HIV diagnoses among young gay men (ages 13-24) of all races and ethnicities rose between 2001 and 2006.[82]

---

74. CDC. HIV/AIDS among Asians and Pacific Islanders. August 2008. Available at http://www.cdc.gov/hiv/resources/factsheets/API.htm

75. CDC. HIV/AIDS among American Indians and Alaska Natives. August 2008. Available at http://www.cdc.gov/hiv/resources/factsheets/aian.htm

76. NASTAD and Kaiser Family Foundation. The National HIV Prevention Inventory: The State of HIV Prevention Across the U.S. July 2009. Available at http://www.kff.org/hivaids/upload/7932.pdf

77. CDC. CDC Fact Sheet: HIV and AIDS among Gay and Bisexual Men. June 2010. Available at http://www.cdc.gov/nchhstp/newsroom/docs/FastFacts-MSM-FINAL508COMP.pdf

78. DW Purcell, C Johnson, A Lansky, et al. Calculating HIV and Syphilis Rates for Risk Groups: Estimating the National Population Size of Men Who Have Sex with Men 2010 National STD Prevention Conference; Atlanta, GA Latebreaker #22896 Presented March 10, 2010.

79. CDC. CDC Fact Sheet: HIV and AIDS among Gay and Bisexual Men. June 2010. Available at http://www.cdc.gov/nchhstp/newsroom/docs/FastFacts-MSM-FINAL508COMP.pdf

80. CDC. HIV/AIDS Surveillance in Urban and Nonurban Areas (through 2007). Available at http://www.cdc.gov/hiv/topics/surveillance/resources/slides/urban-nonurban/index.htm

81. Operario D, Soma T, Underhill K. Sex work and HIV Status among Transgender Women: Systematic Review and Meta-Analysis. *J Acquir Immune Def Syndr* 2008;48(1)97-103.

82. CDC. Trends in HIV/AIDS Diagnoses among men who have sex with men—33 states, 2001-2006. *MMWR* June 2008;57(25):681-686.

Recommended Actions

To refocus our HIV prevention efforts, the following actions are needed:

1.1 **Allocate public funding to geographic areas consistent with the epidemic:** Governments at all levels should ensure that HIV prevention funding is allocated consistent with the latest epidemiological data and is targeted to the highest prevalence populations and communities.

1.2 **Target high-risk populations:** Federal agencies should develop new mechanisms for ensuring that grant funding to State and local health departments and community-based organizations is based on the epidemiological profile within the jurisdiction.

1.2.1 **Prevent HIV among gay and bisexual men and transgender individuals:** Congress and State legislatures should consider the implementation of laws that promote public health practice and underscore the existing best evidence in HIV prevention for sexual minorities.

1.2.2 **Prevent HIV among Black Americans:** To lower risks for all Americans, prevention efforts should acknowledge the heavy burden of HIV among Black Americans and target resources appropriately.

1.2.3 **Prevent HIV among Latino Americans:** HIV prevention efforts that target Latino communities must be culturally appropriate and available to acculturated and non-acculturated Latino populations.

1.2.4 **Prevent HIV among substance users:** Substance use is associated with a greater likelihood of acquiring HIV infection. HIV screening and other comprehensive HIV prevention services should be coupled with substance treatment programs.

1.3 **Address HIV prevention in Asian American and Pacific Islander and American Indian and Alaska Native populations:** Federal and State agencies should consider efforts to support surveillance activities to better characterize HIV among smaller populations such as AAPIs and AI/ANs.

1.4 **Enhance program accountability:** New tools are needed to hold recipients of public funds accountable for achieving results.

Step 2: Expand targeted efforts to prevent HIV infection using a combination of effective, evidence-based approaches.

One of the hardest lessons of the HIV/AIDS epidemic is that there is no single 'magic bullet' that will stem the tide of new HIV infections. In the past, some have focused on one method of HIV prevention in favor of others. The public discourse has over-simplified the policy issues and has led some people to believe that a single solution, whether it is education, condom use, or biomedical innovations, held the key to reducing HIV infections. Our prevention efforts have been hampered by not deploying adequate overlapping, combination approaches to HIV prevention.[83,84] Further, we have not consistently utilized the most effective, cost-efficient tools to prevent HIV or tools that will have a sustainable impact over

83. Auerbach JD, Coates TJ. HIV Prevention Research: Accomplishment and Challenges for the Third decade of AIDS. *Am J Public Health*. 2000;90:1029-1032.

84. UNAIDS. UNAIDS promotes combination HIV prevention towards universal access goals. March 2009. Available at http://www.unaids.org/en/KnowledgeCentre/Resources/PressCentre/PressReleases/2009/20090318_ComprehensivePrevention.asp

the long term.[85] Evaluating and employing multiple scientifically proven methods will have a greater impact to keep people from becoming infected. Additional research can also help identify new prevention strategies and the most effective combination approaches to prevent new HIV infections.

Prevention for people who are HIV-positive is critical to reducing new HIV infections. To prevent HIV, we should strive to ensure that all people living with HIV know their HIV status and are linked to and maintained in high-quality care that includes timely offering of, and promotes adherence to, HIV anti-retroviral therapy, consistent with current clinical practice standards.[86] In addition, all people who are diagnosed with HIV should receive (1) services to assist with notifying recent sex and drug-use partners of the need to get tested for HIV; (2) access to behavioral and biomedical interventions that have been shown to sustainably reduce the probability of transmitting HIV to others and reduce acquisition of other sexually transmitted diseases; and (3) be screened for, and linked to, other medical and social services (as needed, including drug treatment, family planning, housing, and mental health services) that support individuals in reducing their transmission risk.

Moreover, all HIV-negative people at high-risk for HIV infection, especially those in sexual relationships with HIV-positive individuals or those with multiple sex partners, should be tested for HIV and STDs at least once a year. They should also have access to behavioral and biomedical interventions with long-term and sustainable outcomes that reduce the probability of HIV acquisition and also receive other medical and social services (as needed) that reduce the risk of acquiring HIV.

The following are scientifically proven biomedical and behavioral approaches that reduce the probability of HIV transmission:

- **Abstinence from sex or drug use:** Abstaining from sexual activity and substance use reduces the risk of HIV infection. In cases where this may not be possible, limiting the number of partners and taking other steps can lower the risk of acquiring HIV.

- **HIV testing:** There is evidence that people who test HIV-positive take steps to keep others from being exposed to the virus.[87] People who are unaware of their HIV status for an extended period of time may also enter care too late to have the maximum benefit from therapy, and they may unintentionally expose others to HIV.[88]

- **Condom availability:** Condom use is the most effective method to reduce risk of HIV infection during sexual activity. Correct and consistent use of male condoms is estimated to reduce the risk of HIV transmission by 80 percent.[89]

- **Access to sterile needles and syringes:** Among injection drug users, sharing needles and other drug paraphernalia increases the risk of HIV infection. Several studies have found that providing

85. Piot P, Bartos M, Larson H, Zewdie D, Mane P Coming to terms with complexity: a call to action for HIV prevention. *Lancet.*2008 (9641);372:845-859.

86. The National Institutes of Health (NIH) publishes and updates the Department of Health and Human Services clinical practice guidelines for the use of antiretroviral therapy for people living with HIV. The most recent versions of the guidelines for specific populations may be found at http://www.aidsinfo.nih.gov/Guidelines/.

87. Marks G, Crepaz Nicole, Janssen, RS. Estimating sexual transmission of HIV from persons aware and unaware that they are infected with the virus in the USA. *AIDS.*2006;20(10):1447-1450.

88. Bisset L, Cone RW, Huber W, et al. Highly active antiretroviral therapy during early HIV infection reverses T-cell activation and maturation abnormalities. *AIDS* 1998;12(16):2115-23.

89. Weller S, Davis, K. Condom effectiveness in reducing heterosexual HIV transmission (Cochrane Review). In: *The Cochrane Library*, Issue 4, 2003. Chichester, UK: John Wiley & Sons, Ltd.

sterilized equipment to injection drug users substantially reduces risk of HIV infection, increases the probability that they will initiate drug treatment, and does not increase drug use.[90,91]

- **HIV treatment:** In addition to benefiting their own health, studies show that HIV-positive individuals who are adhering to effective antiretroviral therapy are less likely to transmit the virus compared to HIV-positive individuals who are not on medication.[92] There are also specific HIV medications that a person can take immediately after being exposed to HIV that can reduce the risk of HIV infection, called post exposure prophylaxis (PEP).[93] Antiretroviral therapy for pregnant women with HIV also dramatically reduces the risk of HIV transmission during pregnancy and childbirth.[94]

Some other biomedical and behavioral interventions have not been consistently associated with reducing HIV transmission, but may still contribute to our prevention efforts. For example, having an untreated sexually transmitted infection (STI) such as herpes, gonorrhea or syphilis substantially increases a person's chance of acquiring HIV, but research has not yet shown that treating STIs lowers HIV infection at a population level.[95, 96] Nevertheless, all people screened for STIs should also be screened for HIV infection because these infections are driven by the same risk behaviors.[97] Similarly, there are scientifically proven behavioral interventions that reduce HIV risk behaviors such as sexual risk behavior or drug use.[98] Even though these interventions have not been proven to reduce HIV infections, they promote responsible sexual behaviors that may lower a person's risk for becoming infected with HIV and some have been associated with reducing STIs.[99, 100, 101] Not all of the interventions, however, are equally effective over the long-term and not all of them are readily scalable, meaning that they can be effectively and affordably disseminated to large groups of people.[102] Given limited resources and substantial needs in communities heavily impacted by HIV, behavioral interventions that can effectively reach large groups of individuals should be prioritized. Additionally, more operational research is needed to determine which behavioral interventions are scalable and produce robust and sustainable outcomes.

90. Latkin, C, Davey, M, and Hua, W. Needle Exchange Program Utilization and Entry into Drug User Treatment: Is There a Long-Term Connection in Baltimore, Maryland? *Subst Use Misuse*, 41(14):1991-2001.

91. Vlahov D, Junge B. The role of needle exchange programs in HIV prevention. *Public Health Rep*. 1998;113 (Suppl 1):75-80.

92. Donnell D, Baeten JM, Kiarie J, et al. Heterosexual HIV-1 transmission after initiation of antiretroviral therapy: a prospective cohort analysis. *Lancet*. 2010.

93. Smith DK, Grohskopf LA, Black RJ, et al. Antiretroviral postesxposure prophylaxis after sexual, injection-drug use, or other nonoccupational exposure to HIV in the United States. *MMWR*. 2005; 54:1-20.

94. HHS. Recommendations for Use of Antiretroviral Drugs in Pregnant HIV-1 Infected Women for Maternal Health *and* Interventions to Reduce Perinatal HIV Transmission in the United States. May 24, 2010

95. Celum C, Wald A, Hughes J, et al. Effect of acyclovir on HIV-1 acquisition in herpes simplex virus 2 seropositive women and men who have sex with men. *Lancet*. 2008;371:2109-19.

96. Gray RH, Wawer MJ. Reassessing the hypothesis on STI control for Prevention. *Lancet*. 2008; 371(9630): 2064-2065.

97. National Alliance of State and Territorial AIDS Directors, National Coalition of STD Directors. STD/HIV prevention integration; 2002Available from: URL: http://www.ncsddc.org/docs/STDHIVIssuePaperFinal.pdf

98. CDC. 2009 compendium of evidence-based HIV prevention interventions. Available from URL: http://www.cdc.gov/hiv/topics/research/prs/evidence-based-interventions.htm

99. Coates T, Richter L, Caceres C. Behavioural strategies to reduce HIV transmission: how to make them better. *Lancet*. 2008;372(9639):669-684.

100. Koblin B, Chesney M, Coates TJ, for the EXPLORE Study Team. Effects of a behavioural intervention to reduce acquisition of HIV infection among men who have sex with men: the EXPLORE randomised controlled study. *Lancet*. 2004; 364: 41–50.

101. Crepaz N, Horn AK, Rama SM, et al. The efficacy of behavioral interventions in reducing HIV risk sex behaviors and incident sexually transmitted disease in black and Hispanic sexually transmitted disease clinic patients in the United States: a meta-analytic review. *Sex Transm Dis*. 2007;34(6):319-32.

102. Coates T, Richter L, Caceres C. Behavioural strategies to reduce HIV transmission: how to make them better. *Lancet*. 2008;372(9639):669-684.

The quality of information that we have to understand the epidemic we face and how it is changing depends on having an effective HIV surveillance system. The National HIV Surveillance System is the primary source of data used to monitor the epidemic in the United States HIV surveillance data are used extensively to target and evaluate HIV prevention and care programs. Therefore, completeness and timeliness of the data are critical. Surveillance of HIV disease necessitates a complex system of reporting from providers, laboratories, and State and local health departments to coordinate accurate, complete and timely reporting. While the system has performed well, there are few tools to accurately detect people who are newly infected with HIV. This is critical because people who are newly infected with HIV are more infectious than those individuals who have been living with HIV for an extended period of time.[103] Aside from tools to diagnose acute HIV infection, not all HIV surveillance sites track the same key measures in the same way (e.g., viral load, CD4).

Current approaches to preventing HIV must be coupled with research on new and innovative prevention methods that can have a long-term impact. Vaccines and microbicides are two biomedical approaches that are of promising, but safe and effective vaccines and microbicides are not yet available and investments in research to produce safe and effective vaccines and microbicides must continue. In addition, an important area to study is the feasibility and effectiveness of using treatment to prevent new infections. Such strategies include: 1) pre-exposure prophylaxis (PrEP), the use of antiretroviral therapy by high-risk uninfected populations, such as by HIV-negative individuals in committed relationships with HIV-positive individuals; and 2) potential prevention strategies known as 'test and treat' or 'test, treat and link to care' to determine whether a community-wide HIV testing program with an offer of immediate treatment can decrease the overall rate of new HIV infections in that community. Studies are currently underway to test the feasibility of PrEP and 'test and treat' in the United States and multiple sites around the world. Even if these prevention strategies are successful, additional research will be needed to assess the cost effectiveness of these approaches and their adaptability outside of carefully controlled research studies. There will also be a need to couple these approaches with behavioral interventions to ensure that any positive outcomes from PrEP, 'test and treat' or other innovative interventions are not erased by changes in risk behaviors.

There is an opportunity to get better results from our investments in HIV prevention by piloting, evaluating, and expanding access to effective combinations of prevention services.

Recommended Actions

To expand effective approaches to HIV prevention, the following actions are needed:

2.1 **Design and evaluate innovative prevention strategies and combination approaches for preventing HIV in high-risk communities:** Government agencies should fund and evaluate demonstration projects to test which combinations of effective interventions are cost-efficient, produce sustainable outcomes, and have the greatest impact in preventing HIV in specific communities.

---

103. Pilcher CD, Tien HC, Eron JJ, et al. Brief but efficient: Acute HIV infection and the sexual transmission of HIV. *J Infect Dis* 2004; 189(10):1785-1792.

2.2 **Support and strengthen HIV screening and surveillance activities:** There is a need to support existing surveillance methods to identify populations at greatest risk that need to be targeted for HIV prevention services.

2.3 **Expand access to effective prevention services:** Federal funds should support and State and local governments should be encouraged to expand access to effective HIV prevention services with the greatest potential for population-level impact for high-risk populations.

2.4 **Expand prevention with HIV-positive individuals:** Although most people diagnosed with HIV do not transmit the virus to others, there are effective approaches that support people living with HIV in avoiding transmitting HIV to others.

Step 3: Educate all Americans about the threat of HIV and how to prevent it.

If a central tenet of the *National HIV/AIDS Strategy* is that we need to focus our public investments to achieve a maximal response, it is predicated on all Americans having access to a common baseline of information about the current HIV epidemic. This includes knowing how HIV is transmitted and prevented, and knowing which behaviors place individuals at greatest risk for infection. In some communities, many people no longer consider HIV a priority or something that could affect them personally. While we recognize that HIV is concentrated in certain communities, we need to provide all Americans with clear information about how to avoid HIV infection.

Broader HIV education is needed across the age span. Twenty-four percent of people living with HIV are over age 50, and 15 percent of new HIV cases occur in this age group.[104] HIV awareness and education should be universally integrated into all educational environments and health and wellness initiatives. Information about HIV is important to include in any wellness context promoting healthy behaviors, including sexual health. We must also ensure that all health and wellness practitioners (peer counselors, intake specialists, doctors, nurses, and other health professionals) are also educated about HIV, especially in programs for underserved communities. We should ensure that this education reaches populations that may be overlooked, including people with other disabilities. The focus of the education and awareness effort is to improve individual understanding of HIV infection, HIV-related risk factors and risk reduction, and HIV-related stigma and discrimination.

It is also important to educate Americans about how HIV is not transmitted. A significant proportion of the American public harbors misconceptions about how HIV is transmitted. The Kaiser Family Foundation released the results of a survey in 2009, where between one in five or one in ten Americans believed that HIV could be transmitted through sharing a drinking glass, touching a toilet seat, or swimming in a pool with someone who is HIV-positive. Misperceptions varied by demographics and were more common among the elderly, but as many as a third of young people (ages 18-29) held one of these misperceptions. Strikingly, the percentage of the American public that holds these misperceptions has not changed since 1987.[105]

---

104. CDC. HIV/AIDS among Persons Aged 50 and Older. February 2008. Available at
http://www.cdc.gov/hiv/topics/over50/resources/factsheets/over50.htm
105. Kaiser Family Foundation. 2009 Survey of Americans on HIV/AIDS: Summary of Findings on the Domestic Epidemic. Available at http://www.kff.org/kaiserpolls/upload/7889.pdf

Finally, educating young people about HIV before they begin engaging in behaviors that place them at risk for HIV infection should be a priority. Appropriately, it is a parent's job to instill values and to provide the moral and ethical foundation for their children, but schools have an important role in providing access to current and accurate information about the biological and scientific aspects of health education. It is important to provide access to a baseline of health education information that is grounded in the benefits of abstinence and delaying or limiting sexual activity, while ensuring that youth who make the decision to be sexually active have the information they need to take steps to protect themselves.

Recommended Actions

To better educate the American people about HIV/AIDS, the following is needed:

3.1 **Utilize evidence-based social marketing and education campaigns:** Outreach and engagement through traditional media (radio, television, and print) and networked media (such as online health sites, search providers, social media, and mobile applications) must be increased to educate and engage the public about how HIV is transmitted and to reduce misperceptions about HIV transmission. Efforts will be made to utilize and build upon World AIDS Day (December 1st) and National HIV Testing Day (June 27th), as well as other key dates and ongoing activities throughout the year.

3.2 **Promote age-appropriate HIV and STI prevention education for all Americans:** Too many Americans do not have the basic facts about HIV and other sexually transmitted infections. Sustained and reinforcing education is needed to effectively encourage people across the age span to take steps to reduce their risk for infection.

Increasing Access to Care and Improving Health Outcomes for People Living with HIV

Plan to Increase Access to Care and Improve Health Outcomes At-A-Glance

To increase access to care and improve health outcomes, we must work to:

- Establish a seamless system to immediately link people to continuous and coordinated quality care when they are diagnosed with HIV.

- Take deliberate steps to increase the number and diversity of available providers of clinical care and related services for people living with HIV.

- Support people living with HIV with co-occurring health conditions and those who have challenges meeting their basic needs, such as housing.

Anticipated Results:

By 2015:

- Increase the proportion of newly diagnosed patients linked to clinical care within three months of their HIV diagnosis from 65 percent to 85 percent.

- Increase the proportion of Ryan White HIV/AIDS Program clients who are in continuous care (at least 2 visits for routine HIV medical care in 12 months at least 3 months apart) from 73 percent to 80 percent.

- Increase the percentage of Ryan White HIV/AIDS Program clients with permanent housing from 82 percent to 86 percent. (This serves as a measurable proxy of our efforts to expand access to HUD and other housing supports to all needy people living with HIV.)

The Opportunity

While there is not yet a cure for HIV infection, there are a growing number of treatments that can extend life expectancy for those who have access to them. Research remains essential to finding a cure for HIV and to developing safer, more effective therapies and regimens to treat HIV and its associated complications. Access to treatment can be difficult, however, due to the high cost of care which makes insurance coverage a necessity. On average, HIV therapy costs approximately $25,000 per year, and medications are only one portion of a person's total health care needs.[106] Other factors can also prevent people from entering into care and staying on a course of treatment.

Despite our significant public investments in health care services through Medicaid, Medicare, and the Ryan White HIV/AIDS Program, too many people living with HIV do not have access to the medical care that they need. Further, difficult economic times have caused a number of States to reduce or eliminate funding for HIV programs. Waiting lists and other limitations on lifesaving HIV medications are increasing concerns that threaten our progress at getting people with HIV into care.

The *Affordable Care Act*, which will greatly expand access to insurance coverage for people living with HIV, will provide a platform for improvements in health care coverage

---

106. Schackman BR, Gebo KA, Walensky RP, et al. The lifetime cost of current human immunodeficiency virus care in the United States. *Med Care* 2006; 44(11):990-7.

and quality.[107] High risk pools are available immediately. High risk pools will be established in every state to provide coverage to uninsured people with chronic conditions. In 2014, Medicaid will be expanded to all lower income individuals (below 133% of the Federal poverty level, or about $15,000 for a single individual in 2010) under age 65. Uninsured people with incomes up to 400% of the Federal poverty level (about $43,000 for a single individual in 2010) will have access to Federal tax credits and have the opportunity to purchase private insurance coverage through competitive insurance exchanges. New consumer protections will better protect people with private insurance coverage by ending discrimination based on health status and pre-existing conditions. Gaps in essential care and services for people living with HIV will continue to need to be addressed along with the unique biological, psychological, and social effects of living with HIV. As the new law takes effect, it also will be important to ensure that people living with HIV and HIV health care providers are included in the various initiatives that seek to improve the quality of care and integration of services.

The Ryan White HIV/AIDS Program is entering its twentieth year and exists to provide services to the uninsured and to fill in gaps left by private and public insurance coverage. While the program has done impressive work, the level of need has always exceeded available funding. There are ongoing debates about how to fairly allocate limited resources among needy groups or which services to prioritize. Expanded access to insurance coverage will not take care of all needs, but implementation of health insurance reform presents the Nation with an opportunity to re-think what will be needed from the Ryan White HIV/AIDS Program in order to bring people with HIV into care and retain them in care once more people have insurance coverage. Therefore, the Ryan White HIV/AIDS Program and other Federal and State HIV-focused programs will continue to be necessary after the law is implemented to address gaps in essential services for people living with HIV.

People with HIV also have other significant challenges. Many people living with HIV have other co-occurring conditions, such as heart disease, depression or other mental health problems, or drug or alcohol addiction.[108] In addition, poverty, unemployment, domestic violence, homelessness, hunger, lack of access to transportation, and other issues can prevent people from accessing health care. There are also differences in health care access and treatment outcomes by race/ethnicity, gender, and geography. HIV-positive African Americans and Latinos are more likely to die sooner after an AIDS diagnosis compared to HIV-positive Whites; HIV-positive women are less likely to access therapy compared to HIV-positive men; and access to care and supportive services is particularly difficult for HIV-positive persons in rural areas, as well as other underserved communities. [109,110] While research has already brought us a long way, continued research is needed to develop safer, less expensive, and more effective treatments and drug regimens, as well as to evaluate new approaches to meeting HIV treatment needs while also responding to co-occurring conditions or other barriers to care.

---

107. The Patient Protection and *Affordable Care Act* (*Affordable Care Act*), P.L. 111-148 includes numerous provisions that will expand access to insurance coverage for people living with HIV. See, for example, Title II which includes expands Medicaid eligibility and Title I which includes various insurance market reforms.

108. Moore, R.M., Gebo, K.A., Lucas, G.M., Keruly, J.C. Rate of Co-morbidities Not Related to HIV infection or AIDS among HIV-Infected Patients, by CD4 Count and HAART Use Status. *Clin Infect Dis* 2008; 47(8):1102-1104.

109. Hall IH, McDavid K, Ling Q, Sloggett A. Determinants of Progression to AIDS or Death After HIV Diagnosis, United States, 1996 to 2001. *Ann Epidemiol* 2006;16(11): 824-33.

110. Heckman TG, Somlai AM, Peters J, Walker J, Otto-Sajal CA, Galdabni CA, Kelly JA. Barriers to care among persons living with HIV/AIDS in urban and rural areas. *AIDS Care* 1998;10(3):365-75.

To address these issues, we need to expand our approaches to connecting people to services and keeping them in care.

Steps to be Taken

We must pursue a concerted national effort to get and keep people living with HIV in care. The following steps are critical to achieving success:

1. Establish a seamless system to immediately link people to continuous and coordinated quality care when they are diagnosed with HIV.

2. Take deliberate steps to increase the number and diversity of available providers of clinical care and related services for people living with HIV.

3. Support people living with HIV with co-occurring health conditions and those who have challenges meeting their basic needs, such as housing.

Anticipated Results

By 2015

*   Increase the proportion of newly diagnosed patients linked to clinical care within three months of their HIV diagnosis from 65 percent to 85 percent (from 26,824 to 35,079 people).

*   Increase the proportion of Ryan White HIV/AIDS Program clients who are in continuous care (at least 2 visits for routine HIV medical care in 12 months at least 3 months apart) from 73 percent to 80 percent (or 237,924 people in continuous care to 260,739 people in continuous care)

*   Increase the percentage of Ryan White HIV/AIDS Program clients with permanent housing from 82 percent to 86 percent (from 434,000 to 455,800 people). This serves as a measurable proxy of our efforts to expand access to HUD and other housing supports to all needy people living with HIV.

Recommended Actions

Step 1: Establish a seamless system to immediately link people to continuous and coordinated quality care when they learn they are infected with HIV.

Since effective antiretroviral therapies became available in the mid-1990s, questions about when to initiate therapy and how to minimize side effects and complications of long-term medication therapy have been debated. The Federal Government's treatment guidelines, which are the standard of care, have evolved over time and are regularly updated to reflect the most current research findings.[111] While decisions about when to start treatment must remain voluntary and require an individual to be ready to start a long-term regimen, growing evidence suggests that early initiation of treatment leads to improved outcomes.[112] To achieve this clinical goal requires that people are identified soon after their infection and systems are put in place to link them to care. This is particularly important given that over

---

111. The National Institutes of Health (NIH) publishes and updates the Department of Health and Human Services clinical practice guidelines for the use of antiretroviral therapy for people living with HIV. The most recent versions of the guidelines for specific populations may be found at http://www.aidsinfo.nih.gov/Guidelines/.

112. Kitahata MM, Gange SJ, Abraham AG, et al. Effect of early versus deferred antiretroviral therapy for HIV on survival. *New Engl J Med*. 2009; 360(18):1815-1826.

230,000 people living with HIV do not know they are HIV positive, and therefore are not receiving regular medical care to manage the disease.[113]

Since 2006, CDC has recommended routine HIV screening for adults and adolescents ages 13-64 in health care settings. Testing, however, is only one of several critical services needed to get people into care. People who receive a diagnosis of HIV infection need to be connected to appropriate clinical care, prevention, and supportive services. It is essential to provide linkage coordination when and where HIV screening services are provided to help overcome barriers to obtaining care.

One approach to improving linkage to care is co-location of testing and care services. Another approach is using nontraditional sites to provide HIV screening and referral services. A recent study sponsored by the Substance Abuse and Mental Health Services Administration (SAMHSA) indicated that fewer than half of all substance abuse treatment facilities surveyed nationwide reported that they conduct on-site infectious disease screening.[114] Facilities that provided hospital inpatient treatment were more likely than facilities providing only outpatient or nonhospital residential treatment to offer screening for HIV, sexually transmitted diseases (STDs), hepatitis B, hepatitis C, or tuberculosis. Encouraging these types of facilities and nontraditional sites like community centers, mental health centers, or faith institutions to get trained and offer HIV screening and referrals could help build service provider capacity and connect people to the care and treatment they need to address HIV and other co-occurring conditions. This is also one element of a strategy to better meet the HIV prevention and care needs of people living in rural or under-resourced areas. It also provides an opportunity for providers to begin to take a more holistic approach to health, rather than focusing only on HIV. Some of the same behaviors that help to prevent HIV infection also will help to prevent STDs and hepatitis B and C.

Being linked to care is not enough. It is estimated that as many as 30 percent of people diagnosed with HIV are not accessing care. There is a need to re-engage people diagnosed with HIV who have never been in care or who have subsequently fallen out of care. There is also a need for ongoing support to maintain the necessary high levels of adherence to antiretroviral treatment. Government, academic, and pharmaceutical industry research has brought us simpler, more easily tolerated therapies than the initial generation of effective antiretroviral therapies. Safer, more potent, and more durable treatments are still needed. Additionally, we need to better understand how to manage the clinical complications and consequences of HIV infection and long-term use of antiretroviral drugs—including issues related to accelerated heart disease, kidney disease, cancers, and premature aging.[115,116] More work is also needed to understand differences in treatment response between women and men and among racial and ethnic minorities. Public and private insurers and health care providers must also take steps to ensure that all HIV care providers have the knowledge and training to provide quality HIV care consistent with the latest treatment guidelines.

---

113. CDC. HIV prevalence estimates—United States, 2006. *MMWR*. 2008; 57: 1073-1076.

114. SAMHSA. National Survey of Substance Abuse Treatment Services. The N-SSATS Report. February 25, 2010.

115. Aberg JA, Kaplan JE, Libman H, et al. Primary care guidelines for the management of persons infected with human immunodeficiency virus: 2009 update by the HIV Medicine Association of the Infectious Diseases Society of America. *Clin Infect Dis*. 2009;49(5):651-81.

116. DHHS Panel on Antiretroviral Guidelines for Adults and Adolescents. Guidelines for the use of antiretroviral agents in HIV-1-infected adults and adolescents. Department of Health and Human Services. December 1, 2009; 1-161. Available at http://www.aidsinfo.nih.gov/ContentFiles/AdultandAdolescentGL.pdf

Recommended Actions

To put this key action step into practice, the following are needed:

1.1 **Facilitate linkages to care:** HIV resources should be targeted to include support for linkage coordinators in a range of settings where at risk populations receive health and social services.

1.2 **Promote collaboration among providers:** All levels of government should increase collaboration between HIV medical care providers and agencies providing HIV counseling and testing services, mental health treatment, substance abuse treatment, housing and supportive services to link people with HIV to care.

1.3 **Maintain people living with HIV in care:** Clinical care providers should ensure that all eligible HIV-positive persons have access to antiretroviral therapy. Those who start therapy need to be maintained on a medication regimen, as recommended by the HHS treatment guidelines.

Step 2: Take deliberate steps to increase the number and diversity of available providers of clinical care and related services for people living with HIV.

To improve health outcomes, we need to adopt policies that will produce a workforce that is large enough to care for all people living with HIV, is diverse, has the appropriate training and technical expertise to provide high-quality care consistent with the latest treatment guidelines, and has the capacity, through shared experiences or training, to provide care in a non-stigmatizing manner and create relationships of trust with their patients. Specialized HIV care should also incorporate prevention. Efforts to expand the HIV workforce of highly skilled professionals should target the areas where the need is greatest.

For too long, our nation has suffered from a severe shortage of primary care health professionals. The *Affordable Care Act* provides for significant new policies and resources to begin to address these issues. In addition, the provider workforce of physicians, nurses, and other health professionals that specialize in HIV care is aging, and new recruits are needed to address the workforce shortage. According to the Association of American Medical Colleges, nearly one fourth (24.7 percent) of the active physician workforce in the United States was age 60 or older in 2008.[117] Within a medical specialty like infectious disease, the problem of limited physician supply is more pronounced. The *Affordable Care Act* and its investments in the National Health Service Corps will help to alleviate primary care workforce shortages in underserved areas, but it is also necessary to encourage more health care providers, including nonphysician providers, to obtain specialized HIV training and include people living with HIV in their practices. Surveys by HIV provider associations indicate that the pending shortage of HIV providers and the increases in HIV patient loads during recent years require an urgent response in order to maintain a robust HIV care system in the United States.[118] Specialized training, task shifting and use of interdisciplinary health teams all can help alleviate HIV workforce shortages. Providers should also consider including peer-based programming, such as peer treatment educators, to reduce workforce burden and to help retain HIV-positive people, especially among hard-to-reach populations, in care.

---

117. Association of American Medical Colleges. 2009 State Physician Workforce Data Book. November 2009.

118. AAHIVM and HIVMA Medical Workforce Working Group. Averting a Crisis in HIV Care: A Joint Statement of the American Academy of HIV Medicine (AAHIVM) and the HIV Medicine Association (HIVMA) on the HIV Medical Workforce. June 2009.

Enhanced program integration is another approach that can be useful in expanding the workforce of professionals providing HIV services. For example, by integrating HIV screening along with reproductive health care, it is possible to effectively address concurrent sexually transmitted infections (STIs), which increase risk for HIV transmission. Providing better integrated, coordinated care will help ensure individuals receive services to prevent and treat opportunistic infections and have their other chronic health needs met, ultimately leading to improved health outcomes and better quality of life.

Strategies available to increase the number of HIV providers include health professions training grants, the National Health Service Corps Scholarship and Loan Repayment Programs, financial incentives to compensate providers for HIV care management, and program coordination so that providers who are not HIV specialists are adequately equipped to provide prevention services to high-risk populations and link patients who test positive to HIV clinical care providers. For example, substance abuse treatment providers may not be HIV specialists, but their patient population may be engaging in behaviors that put them at risk for HIV infection. Therefore, substance abuse and mental health treatment providers are potential providers of HIV prevention services. Oral health care plays an important role because HIV disease can cause certain symptoms identifiable only through dental exams. Dental care providers who are educated about HIV can be referral sources to other services that people living with HIV may need. Similarly, gynecologists and family planning services can be a source of HIV prevention services for women who may or may not be engaging in high-risk behaviors, but who might not actively seek services from an HIV or sexually transmitted disease clinic. Over 70 percent of women ages 15-44 received at least one family planning or medical care service from a medical care provider in the last 12 months.[119] Increasing the number of HIV providers, as well as increasing knowledge among all health professionals about HIV risks and prevention is a critical need. This involves a wide range of health professionals in all health care settings including physicians, registered nurses, nurse practitioners, physician assistants, social workers, pharmacists, and dentists.

Health care services that are respectful of and responsive to the health beliefs, practices and cultural and linguistic needs of diverse patients can help bring about positive health outcomes.[120] Many people living with HIV come from communities that have been historically poorly served by the mainstream health care system. For example, among some African Americans, there is mistrust of the medical establishment, and it may lead some to question clinical recommendations that are widely accepted by others.[121] Heterosexual providers may not be comfortable asking about sexual history when taking a patient's history and this may limit appropriate care.[122] Transgender individuals are particularly challenged in finding providers who respect them and with whom they can have honest discussions about hormone use and other practices, and this results in lower satisfaction with their care providers, less trust, and poorer health outcomes.[123] Findings from an AHRQ-funded study indicated that poor health literacy among people with living with HIV negatively impacts their adherence to antiretroviral medications and their health outcomes.[124] In addition to having HIV expertise, care providers should be

---

119. CDC. National Survey of Family Growth. Available at http://www.cdc.gov/nchs/nsfg/abc_list.htm

120. AHRQ. 2009 *National Healthcare Quality Report*. March 2010.

121. Cargill VA, Stone VE. HIV/AIDS: a minority health issue. *Med Clin North Am* 200;89(4):895-912.

122. Solursh DS, Ernst JL, Lewis RW et al. The human sexuality education of physicians in North American Schools. *Int J Imp Res* 2003;15(Suppl 5):S41-5.

123. Williamson C.. Providing care to transgender persons: a clinical approach to primary care, hormones, and HIV management. *J Assoc Nurses AIDS Care* 2010;21(3):221-229.

124. Kalichman SC, Ramachandran B, Catz S. Adherence to combination antiretroviral therapies in HIV patients of low health literacy. *J Gen Intern Med* 1999;14(5):267-73

culturally competent and able to clearly and effectively communicate to help their patients understand the benefits of following treatment plans.

Recommended Actions

To put this key action step into practice, the following are needed:

> **2.1** **Increase the number of available providers of HIV care:** Federal agencies should develop strategies for encouraging more clinicians including primary care providers, reproductive health care providers and sexually transmitted disease experts, mental health providers, and substance abuse treatment professionals to provide HIV services.

> **2.2** **Strengthen the current provider workforce to improve quality of HIV care and health outcomes for people living with HIV:** Federal agencies should engage clinical providers and professional medical societies on the importance of routine, voluntary HIV screening and quality HIV care in clinical settings consistent with CDC guidelines.

Step 3: Support people living with HIV with co-occurring health conditions and those who have challenges meeting their basic needs, such as housing.

To support the provision of quality care for people living with HIV, it is important to reduce barriers that impede access to services. The concept of a medical home is a model for the provision of coordinated, person-centered care for individuals with chronic or prolonged illnesses requiring regular medical monitoring, care management, and treatment. The Ryan White HIV/AIDS Program has supported the development of medical homes for people living with HIV and has experience to share, which can be valuable to other providers including community health centers and private physicians in their provision of HIV care.[125]

Chronic diseases like heart disease, cancer, and diabetes are leading causes of death and disability in the United States. Many people with HIV have these and other chronic conditions, such as hepatitis, diabetes, and mental illness. Co-infection with other sexually transmitted infections like herpes, syphilis and gonorrhea is also common. It is estimated that up to 50 percent of people with HIV have a mental illness such as depression, and 13 percent have both mental illness and substance abuse issues.[126] Co-infection with HIV and Hepatitis C occurs in 50-90 percent of HIV-infected injection drug users.[127] As people age, the likelihood of having multiple chronic illnesses increases, even among people who do not have HIV. HIV disease itself, as well as long-term use of HIV therapies may also contribute to common chronic conditions, such as heart disease and kidney disease.[128] Additional research is needed to better understand, prevent, and treat these co-infections and complications of HIV disease.

Optimal clinical care should include a range of integrated clinical and preventive services to reduce HIV-related morbidity and mortality. Patient-centered care–defined by the Institute of Medicine as health care that establishes a partnership among practitioners, patients, and their families (when appropriate)

---

125. Saag MS. Ryan White: An Unintentional Home Builder. *AIDS Reader* 2009; 19:166-168.

126. Bing EG, Burnman MA, Longshore D, et al. Psychiatric disorders and drug use among human immunodeficiency virus-infected adults in the United States. *Arch Gen Psych* 2001 58(8):721-728.

127. CDC Fact Sheet. Coinfection with HIV and Hepatitis C Virus. November 2005. Available at http://www.cdc.gov/hiv/resources/factsheets/coinfection.htm

128. El-Sadr WM, Lundgren JD, Neaton JD, et a. Strategies for Management of Antiretroviral Therapy (SMART) Study Group. CD4+ count-guided interruption of antiretroviral treatment. *N Engl J Med* 2001,355(22):2283-2296.

to ensure that decisions respect patients' wants, needs, and preferences–should be the standard. In addition to ensuring that clinical care services are well coordinated, non-medical services and assistance to meet basic needs are important supports for achieving good clinical outcomes. Access to medical treatment should be supplemented with ongoing case management services to facilitate continuity of care. Supportive services such as transportation, legal assistance, nutrition services, mental health services, substance use treatment, and child care are essential for certain populations facing difficulties with everyday needs.

Access to housing is an important precursor to getting many people into a stable treatment regimen. Individuals living with HIV who lack stable housing are more likely to delay HIV care, have poorer access to regular care, are less likely to receive optimal antiretroviral therapy, and are less likely to adhere to therapy. A large-scale study from 2007 comparing the health of homeless and stably housed people living with HIV found that housing status was more significant than individual characteristics as a pre-dictor of health care access and outcomes.[129] A long-term study of people living with HIV in New York City found that over a 12-year period, receipt of housing assistance was one of the strongest predictors of accessing HIV primary care, maintaining continuous care, receiving care that meets clinical practice standards, and entry into HIV care.[130] Receipt of housing assistance had a direct impact on improved medical care, regardless of demographics, drug use, health and mental health status, or receipt of other services. *Opening Doors: Federal Strategic Plan to Prevent and End Homelessness* focuses efforts to reduce homelessness and increase housing security. Planning efforts will be undertaken in collaboration with community partners to address the housing needs of vulnerable Americans who are in homeless situ-ations or present risks of homelessness.

People with competing demands and challenges meeting their basic needs for housing, food, and child care often have problems staying in care. Access to legal services can be important to help people resolve issues with discrimination, access to public benefits including health care, and resolving prob-lems with employment and other issues that can create serious barriers to staying in care. Support from social workers and/or case managers can help with identifying resources, and peer networks among people living with HIV may also be valuable for information sharing and other support. Programs that provide family-centered care can be especially important for women living with HIV. Further, both women and men with HIV can be at risk for intimate partner violence, which can impede adherence and stability in care. As HIV service providers develop ways to improve delivery of care for these and other specific populations, including youth, people in or transitioning from correctional settings, and people living in remote or rural areas, it will be important to disseminate information about effective models to enable other providers to better serve those groups and overcome common barriers to care.

129. Kidder DP, Wolitski RJ, Campsmith,ML, Nakamura, GV. Health status, health care use, medication use, and medication adherence in homeless and housed people living with HIV/AIDS. *Am J Public Health.* 2007; 97(12):2238-2245.

130. Aidala, AA, Lee, G, Abramson, DM, Messeri, P, Siegler, A. Housing need, housing assistance, and connection to medical care. *AIDS Behav* 2007;11(Supp 2): S101-S115.

Recommended Actions

To put this key action step into practice, the following are needed:

3.1 **Enhance client assessment tools and measurement of health outcomes:** Federal and State agencies should support case management and clinical services that contribute to improving health outcomes for people living with HIV and work toward increasing access to non-medical supportive services (e.g., housing, food, transportation) as critical elements of an effective HIV care system.

3.2 **Address policies to promote access to housing and supportive services for people living with HIV:** Federal agencies should consider additional efforts to support housing assistance and other services that enable people living with HIV to obtain and adhere to HIV treatment.

Reducing HIV-Related Disparities
and Health Inequities

Plan to Reduce HIV-Related Disparities and Health Inequities At-A-Glance

Disparities in HIV prevention and care persist among racial/ethnic minorities, as well as among sexual minorities. While working to improve access to prevention and care services for all Americans, the following steps will help to reduce inequities across groups:

- Reduce HIV-related mortality in communities at high risk for HIV infection.

- Adopt community-level approaches to reduce HIV infection in high-risk communities.

- Reduce stigma and discrimination against people living with HIV.

Anticipated Results:

By 2015:

- Increase the proportion of HIV diagnosed gay and bisexual men with undetectable viral load by 20 percent.

- Increase the proportion of HIV diagnosed Blacks with undetectable viral load by 20 percent.

- Increase the proportion of HIV diagnosed Latinos with undetectable viral load by 20 percent.

The Opportunity

The transmission of HIV has long been concentrated in groups that have been marginalized or underserved.[131] For persons living with HIV, this issue often transcends discrete measures such as incidence, morbidity and mortality rates, but speaks to a confluence of factors that lead to poorer health overall. In some communities, a major challenge is overcoming a sense of fatalism where people believe that they are destined to become infected with HIV. In other communities, although the threat of HIV is real, it is only one of many issues individuals face on a daily basis and may rank lower than more immediate needs such as shelter, food, or safety. In still other communities, people may want to prioritize HIV prevention and care, but services are not easily accessible to them. A national response to the HIV epidemic needs to be mindful of the size, diversity and richness of our country, as well as the needs of the most affected communities.

HIV exists within a health care system where different groups have varying access to services—and achieve varying health outcomes. The *Affordable Care Act* represents the broadest Federal effort, to date, to address health inequities. The law says that a group is a health disparity population when:

"there is a significant disparity in the overall rate of disease incidence, prevalence, morbidity, mortality, or survival rates in the population as compared to the health status of the general population." In addition, it may be determined, "that such term includes populations for which there is a significant disparity in the quality, outcomes, cost, or use of healthcare services or access to or satisfaction with such services as compared to the general population."

By greatly expanding access to health care for all, taking specific steps to support treatment adherence for people

---

131. El-Sadr W, Mayer KH, Hodder SL. AIDS in America—Forgotten but not Gone. *New Engl J Med.* 2010.

living with HIV, conducting research on the causes of differences in health outcomes, and refocusing our prevention efforts on combination strategies targeted to the highest risk communities, we will create the conditions where serious progress can be made in reducing HIV-related health disparities. What is missing are community-level approaches to altering the conditions in which HIV is transmitted and addressing the factors that influence disparate health outcomes among people living with HIV, including lessening stigma and discrimination.

Steps To Be taken

A concerted national effort to increase the capacity of whole communities to prevent HIV and support community members living with HIV is needed. The following steps are critical to achieving success:

1. Reduce HIV-related mortality in communities at high risk for HIV infection.

2. Adopt community-level approaches to reduce HIV infection in high-risk communities.

3. Reduce stigma and discrimination against people living with HIV.

Anticipated Results

By 2015

- Increase the proportion of HIV diagnosed gay and bisexual men with undetectable viral load by 20 percent.

- Increase the proportion of HIV diagnosed Blacks with undetectable viral load by 20 percent.

- Increase the proportion of HIV diagnosed Latinos with undetectable viral load by 20 percent.

Recommended Actions

Step 1: Reduce HIV-related mortality in communities at high risk for HIV infection.
Significant racial disparities in HIV infection exist in the United States (Figure 4). According to CDC, the overall rate of HIV diagnosis for Blacks was roughly eight times the rate for Whites in 2006. The HIV diagnosis rate for all Black males (119.1 per 100,000 population) remains the highest of any racial/ethnic group and is more than seven times that for White males, twice the rate for Latino males, and twice the rate for Black females.[132] Additionally, the diagnosis rate for Latino males was approximately three times that for White males. The HIV diagnosis rate in 2006 for Black females and Latinas was more than 19 times and 5 times (respectively) the rate for White females. Disparities in HIV infection also exist between gay and bisexual men and heterosexual populations. Recently, the CDC announced that gay and bisexual men in the United States are 44 to 86 times more likely to become infected with HIV than heterosexual men, and 40 to 77 times more likely to become infected than women.[133]

---

132. CDC. HIV and AIDS in the United States: A Picture of Today's Epidemic. 2008. Available at http://www.cdc.gov/hiv/topics/surveillance/united_states.htm

133. DW Purcell, C Johnson, A Lansky, et al. Calculating HIV and Syphilis Rates for Risk Groups: Estimating the National Population Size of Men Who Have Sex with Men 2010 National STD Prevention Conference; Atlanta, GA Latebreaker #22896 Presented March 10, 2010.

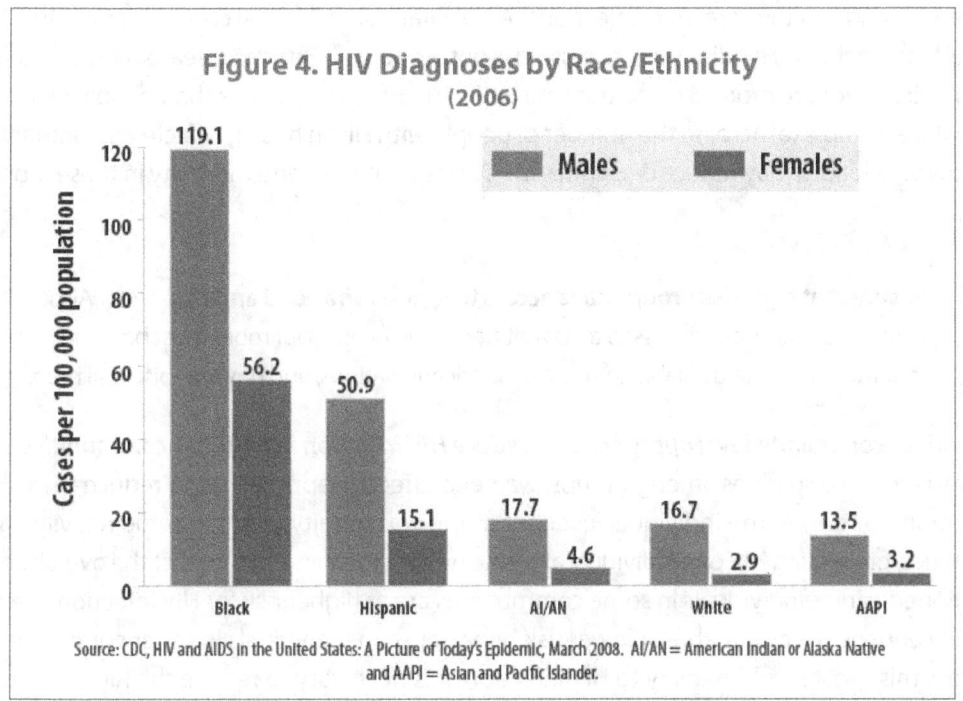

Figure 4. HIV Diagnoses by Race/Ethnicity (2006)

Source: CDC, HIV and AIDS in the United States: A Picture of Today's Epidemic, March 2008. AI/AN = American Indian or Alaska Native and AAPI = Asian and Pacific Islander.

Unfortunately, these disparities in HIV infection also translate into disparities in premature death. Even though HIV-related mortality has been declining since the availability of effective medications, Black and Latino Americans are more likely than White Americans to die earlier from AIDS.[134] Racial disparities in HIV-related deaths also exist among gay men, where Black and Latino gay men are more likely to die from AIDS compared to White men, and among women with Black women and Latinas at greater risk for death compared to White women.[135,136] Gay and bisexual men comprise the majority of people with HIV who have died in the United States.[137]

Decisions about when to start therapies for HIV are personal. There is accumulating scientific evidence, however, that early initiation of antiretroviral therapy improves health outcomes among people living with HIV.[138,139] To achieve these results, it is necessary for people on therapy to be adherent to their medication regimen. Antiretroviral therapy reduces the amount of virus in the bloodstream and improves the health of people living with HIV, in addition to reducing the transmissibility of HIV. A key indicator for health and transmissibility is viral load, which is a way of measuring the amount of virus in a person's body. A high viral load (5,000 to 10,000 copies per milliliter of blood) means that a person's HIV disease

134. Losina E, Schackman BR, Sadownik SN, et al. Racial and Sex Disparities in Life Expectancy Losses among HIV-Infected Persons in the United States. *Clin Infect Dis* 2009;49(10):1570-8.

135. Hall HI, Byers RH, Ling Q, Espinoza L. Racial/Ethnic and Age Disparities in HIV Prevalence and Disease Progression Among Men Who Have Sex With Men in the United States. *Am J Public Health*. 2007;97(6):1060-66

136. Losina E, Schackman BR, Sadownik SN, et al. Racial and Sex Disparities in Life Expectancy Losses among HIV-Infected Persons in the United States. *Clin Infect Dis* 2009;49(10):1570-8.

137. CDC. HIV in the United States: An overview. June 2010. Available at http://www.cdc.gov/hiv/topics/surveillance/resources/factsheets/us_overview.htm

138. Quinn TC, Wawer MJ, Sewankambo N, et al. Viral Load and Heterosexual Transmission of Human Immunodeficiency Virus Type 1. *New Engl J Med* 2000;342(13):921-29.

139. Donnell D, Baeten JM, Kiarie J, et al. Heterosexual HIV-1 transmission after initiation of antiretroviral therapy: a prospective cohort analysis. *Lancet* 2010;375(9731):2092-8.

is progressing and that they are more infectious. A low viral load (40 to 500 copies per milliliter of blood) indicates that a person's HIV disease progression is not as rapid.[140] Besides disease progression, people with high viral loads are more likely to transmit HIV to uninfected partners than people with low viral loads.[141] If we are able to increase the number of people with HIV in heavily affected communities who have a low viral load, it may reduce disparities in HIV infection rates and mortality in these groups.

Recommended Actions

1.1   **Ensure that high-risk groups have access to regular viral load and CD4 tests:** All persons living with HIV should have access to tests that track their health, but more must be done to make sure that these tests are available to African Americans, Latinos, and gay and bisexual men.

Step 2: Adopt community-level approaches to reduce HIV infection in high-risk communities.
In order to reduce disparities among groups, we need effective approaches to reduce the risk of HIV transmission not only at the individual level but at the community level. In some heavily impacted communities, preventing HIV one individual at a time will not meaningfully impact the overall epidemic. As mentioned earlier, individuals in some communities are at higher risk for HIV infection even if they personally engage in comparable or lower risk behavior than individuals in other communities.[142,143] To address this greater vulnerability to HIV infection, it is necessary to reduce the high proportion of individuals in these communities who are living with HIV. The viral load of a person living with HIV is associated with transmissibility. Moreover, the scientific evidence shows that the average viral load among all diagnosed HIV-positive individuals in a given community who are in care is strongly associated with the number of new infections that occur in that community.[144,145] Thus, neighborhoods with a high community viral load are also places where uninfected individuals are at greater risk for acquiring HIV than neighborhoods or other localities with a comparatively lower viral load. Innovative solutions such as reducing community viral load may help reduce the number of new HIV infections in specific communities that may, in turn, reduce disparities in HIV infection.[116] Recently, NIH has launched a pilot study in Washington, D.C., and is working with CDC to launch a companion study in the Bronx, New York, to test this approach.[147]

HIV is often only one of many conditions that plague communities at greater risk for HIV infection. In many cases, it is not possible to effectively address HIV transmission or care without also addressing

140. Sterling TR, Vlahov D, Astemborski J, et al. Initial Plasma HIV-1 RNA levels and progression to AIDS in women and men. *New Engl J Med* 2001; 344(10):720-725.

141. Donnell D, Baeten JM, Kiarie J, et al. Heterosexual HIV-1 transmission after initiation of antiretroviral therapy: a prospective cohort analysis. *Lancet* 2010;375(9731):2092-8.

142. Millett GA, Flores SA, Peterson J, Bakeman R. Explaining disparities in HIV infection among Black and White men who have sex with men: A meta-analysis of HIV risk behaviors. *AIDS* 2007;21(15): 2083-2091.

143. Hallfors DD, Iritani BJ, Miller WC, Bauer DJ. Sexual and Drug Behavior Patterns and HIV/STD Racial Disparities: The Need for New Directions. *Am J Public Health.* 2007;97(1):125-132.

144. Das M, Chu PL, Santos G-M, Scheer S, Vittinghoff E, et al. 2010 Decreases in Community Viral Load Are Accompanied by Reductions in New HIV Infections in San Francisco. *PLoS ONE* 5(6): e11068. doi:10.1371/journal.pone.0011068.

145. Wood E, Kerr T, Marshall BDL, et al. Longitudinal community plasma HIV-1 RNA concentrations and incidence of HIV-1 among injecting drug users: prospective cohort study. *BMJ.* 2009;338:b1649.

146. Montaner J et al. *Association of expanded HAART coverage with a decrease in new HIV diagnoses, particularly among injection drug users in British Columbia, Canada.* 17th Conference on Retroviruses and Opportunistic Infections, San Francisco, abstract 88LB, 2010.

147. NIH Press Release: NIH and D.C. Department of Health Team up to Combat District's HIV/AIDS Epidemic, January 12, 2010. Available at http://www.nih.gov/news/health/jan2010/niaid-12.htm

sexually transmitted diseases, substance use, poverty, homelessness and other issues.[148,149] For example, a recent study found that hunger was associated with poor viral suppression among homeless and marginally housed HIV-positive adults taking antiretroviral therapy.[150] Because of these many co-occurring issues, it is important to employ a holistic approach to HIV prevention and care that extends beyond risk behaviors of the individual and address not only mental health, but contextual factors such as sexual and drug use networks, joblessness or homelessness and others that increase risk for infection or suboptimal access or response to care. Although there have been some successful efforts in this regard, such as interventions that examine the link between homelessness and HIV risk behavior, there are too few proven models associated with reducing HIV incidence or increasing access to care that have had a community-level impact.

Recommended Actions

To achieve a community-level impact at lowering HIV infections, the following actions are needed:

    2.1   **Establish pilot programs that utilize community models:** In order to reduce disparities between various groups affected by the epidemic, testing community-level approaches is needed to identify effective interventions that reduce the risk of infection in high prevalence communities.

    2.2   **Measure and utilize community viral load:** Ensure that all high prevalence localities are able to collect data necessary to calculate community viral load, measure the viral load in specific communities, and reduce viral load in those communities where HIV incidence is high.

    2.3   **Promote a more holistic approach to health:** Promote a more holistic approach to health that addresses not only HIV prevention among African Americans, Latinos, gay and bisexual men, women, and substance users, but also the prevention of HIV related co-morbidities, such as STDs and hepatitis B and C.

Step 3: Reduce stigma and discrimination against people living with HIV.
In the earliest days of the HIV epidemic, fear, ignorance, and denial led to harsh, ugly treatment of people living with the disease, and some Americans even called for forced quarantine of all people living with HIV.[151] Although such extreme measures never occurred, the stigma and discrimination faced by people living with HIV was often extremely high. Even today, some people living with HIV still face discrimination in many areas of life including employment, housing, provision of health care services, and access to public accommodations. This undermines efforts to encourage all people to learn their HIV status, and it makes it harder for people to disclose their HIV status to their medical providers, their sex partners, and even clergy and others from whom they may seek understanding and support.

Time and again, an essential element of what has caused social attitudes to change has been when the public sees and interacts with people who are openly living with HIV. For decades, community

148. Holtgrave DR, Crosby RA. Social capital, poverty, and income inequality as predictors of gonorrhoea, syphilis, chlamydia and AIDS case rates in the United States. *Sex Transm Infect.* 2003;79(1):62-64.

149. Stall R, Mills TC, Williamson J, et al. Association of Co-Occurring Psychosocial Health Problems and Increased Vulnerability to HIV/AIDS Among Urban Men Who Have Sex With Men. *Am J Public Health.* 2003;93(6):939-942.

150. Weiser SD, Frongillo EA, Ragland K, Hogg RS, Riley ED, Bangsberg DR. Food insecurity is associated with incomplete HIV RNA suppression among homeless and marginally housed HIV-infected individuals in San Francisco. *J Gen Internal Med* 2009; 24(1):14-20.

151. National Library of Medicine. Profiles in Science: Visual Culture and Health - HIV/AIDS. 2003.

organizations have operated speakers bureaus where people with HIV go into schools, businesses, and churches to talk about living with HIV. In the 1990s, both major political parties had memorable keynote speakers at their presidential nominating conventions that were living with HIV.[152] We know that many people feel shame and embarrassment when they learn their HIV status. And, there is too much social stigma that seeks to assign blame to people who acquire HIV. Encouraging more individuals to disclose their HIV status directly lessens the stigma associated with HIV. As we promote disclosure, however, we must also ensure that we are protecting people who are openly living with HIV. This calls for a continued commitment to civil rights enforcement.

This year marks the twentieth anniversary of the *Americans with Disabilities Act*, the landmark civil rights law that has proven so vital to the protection of people with disabilities including HIV. To be free of discrimination on the basis of HIV status is both a human and a civil right. Vigorous enforcement of the *Americans with Disabilities Act*, the *Fair Housing Act*, the *Rehabilitation Act*, and other civil rights laws is vital to establishing an environment where people will feel safe in getting tested and seeking treatment. Recently, the Obama Administration completed the process begun in the Bush Administration to eliminate the HIV entry ban that restricted noncitizens living with HIV from entering the United States. These and other policy actions have been positive steps forward in lessening the stigma associated with living with HIV.

Working to end the stigma and discrimination experienced by people living with HIV is a critical component of curtailing the epidemic. The success of public health policy depends upon the cooperation of the affected populations. People at high risk for HIV cannot be expected to, nor will they seek testing or treatment services if they fear that it would result in adverse consequences of discrimination. HIV stigma has been shown to be a barrier to HIV testing and people living with HIV who experience more stigma have poorer physical and mental health and are more likely to miss doses of their medication.[153]

An important step we can take is to ensure that laws and policies support our current understanding of best public health practices for preventing and treating HIV. At least 32 states have HIV-specific laws that criminalize behavior by people living with HIV.[154] Some criminalize behavior like spitting and biting by people with HIV, and were initially enacted at a time when there was less knowledge about HIV's transmissibility. Since it is now clear that spitting and biting do not pose significant risks for HIV transmission, many believe that it is unfair to single out people with HIV for engaging in these behaviors and should be dealt with in a consistent manner without consideration of HIV status. Some laws criminalize consensual sexual activity between adults on the basis that one of the individuals is a person with HIV who failed to disclose their status to their partner. CDC data and other studies, however, tell us that intentional HIV transmission is atypical and uncommon.[155] A recent research study also found that HIV-specific laws do not influence the behavior of people living with HIV in those states where these laws exist.[156] While we understand the intent behind such laws, they may not have the desired effect and they may make people less willing to disclose their status by making people feel at even greater risk of

---

152. In 1992, Bob Hattoy addressed the Democratic National Convention and Mary Fischer addressed the Republican National Convention, and both openly acknowledged living with HIV.

153. Valdiserri, RO. HIV/AIDS stigma: an impediment to public health. *Am J Public Health* 2002;92(3):341-342.

154. Kaiser Family Foundation. Criminal statutes on HIV transmission. 2008. Available at http://www.statehealthfacts.org/comparetable.jsp?ind=569&cat=11

155. CDC. HIV Prevention in the United States at a Critical Crossroads. 2009. Available at http://www.cdc.gov/hiv/resources/reports/pdf/hiv_prev_us.pdf

156. Horvath KJ, Weinmeyer R, Rosser S. An examination of attitudes among US men who have sex with men and the impact of state law. *AIDS Care*. 2010 (in press)

discrimination. In some cases, it may be appropriate for legislators to reconsider whether existing laws continue to further the public interest and public health. In many instances, the continued existence and enforcement of these types of laws run counter to scientific evidence about routes of HIV transmission and may undermine the public health goals of promoting HIV screening and treatment.[157,158]

Recommended Actions

To reduce stigma and discrimination experienced by people living with HIV, the following are needed:

3.1 **Engage communities to affirm support for people living with HIV:** Faith communities, businesses, schools, community-based organizations, social gathering sites, and all types of media outlets should take responsibility for affirming nonjudgmental support for people living with HIV and high-risk communities.

3.2 **Promote public leadership of people living with HIV:** Governments and other institutions (including HIV prevention community planning groups and Ryan White planning councils and consortia) should work with people with AIDS coalitions, HIV services organizations, and other institutions to actively promote public leadership by people living with HIV.

3.3 **Promote public health approaches to HIV prevention and care:** State legislatures should consider reviewing HIV-specific criminal statutes to ensure that they are consistent with current knowledge of HIV transmission and support public health approaches to preventing and treating HIV.

3.4 **Strengthen enforcement of civil rights laws:** The Department of Justice and Federal agencies must enhance cooperation to facilitate enforcement of Federal antidiscrimination laws.

157. Burris S, Cameron E. *The case against criminalization of HIV transmission.* JAMA. 2008;300(5): 578-581.
158. UNAIDS. Criminal law, public health and HIV transmission: A policy options paper. June 2002. Available at http://data.unaids.org/publications/IRC-pub02/jc733-criminallaw_en.pdf

Achieving a More Coordinated National Response to the HIV Epidemic

Plan to Achieve a More Coordinated National Response to the HIV Epidemic in the United States At-A-Glance

In order for the *National HIV/AIDS Strategy* to be successful, emphasis must be placed on coordination of activities among agencies and across all levels of government.

- Increase the coordination of HIV programs across the Federal Government and between Federal agencies and State, territorial, local, and tribal governments.

- Develop improved mechanisms to monitor and report on progress toward achieving national goals.

The Opportunity

The United States does many things right in how it responds to HIV. Persistent advocacy, research accomplishments, and observable successes in preventing HIV and providing health care and social supports to people with HIV have left us with a legacy of global leadership. We have also learned important lessons about how to engage affected communities and how to mobilize broad sectors of society to care about a condition that is highly stigmatized, associated with sexuality, drug use, and other issues that magnify our cultural divides. The United States investment in responding to the domestic HIV epidemic has risen to more than $19 billion per year.[159] This number alone says nothing about whether it is sufficient to meet existing needs or if these resources are used most effectively–and we believe that evaluation of existing funds along with increased investments in certain key areas are warranted. Nonetheless, it is clear that the Nation has devoted significant financial resources to mount a serious and sustained response to ending the HIV epidemic.

What has been missing and what is needed at this time is an enhanced focus on coordinating our efforts across Federal agencies, across all levels of government, with external partners, and throughout the health care system. Further, with dispersed responsibility for responding to HIV, there is a need for a clearer understanding of roles and increased accountability. Since our ultimate success at ending the HIV epidemic depends on the American people understanding the urgency of the challenge and remaining supportive of the important investments we are making in research, care, and prevention, a greater priority should be placed on communicating to the public the challenges we face and the progress we are making.

The many Federal agencies that operate critical HIV programs operate under their own statutory authority as established by Congress. It is not possible or desirable to merge all HIV programs under one roof. At the same time, improved coordination is possible and we can improve the Federal response by insisting that agencies work in closer collaboration with each other.

---

159. FY 2010 Appropriations.

In our Federal system, the role of the Federal Government is not to direct all activities by all entities. Indeed, in our diverse country, the most effective responses are often those that originate at the State or local level, or even at the level of individual neighborhoods. In this environment, Federal leadership is critical in identifying overarching national priorities, as well as supporting research to evaluate which activities are most effective and then ensuring that Federal resources are deployed to maximal effect. Many Federal HIV prevention and care programs operate largely by providing resources to State, local and tribal governments to provide services within Federal rules and guidelines. While flexibility is critical to respond to varied needs, our three decades of experience of fighting HIV has given the Nation a greater sense of what is effective. Therefore, it is appropriate for the Federal Government to focus the use of its resources on tools that have been shown to work effectively in addressing the Administration's *National HIV/AIDS Strategy* goals and to prioritize the utilization of epidemiological data in the policy-making process.

Much can be achieved by prioritizing enhanced collaboration and accountability.

Steps to be Taken

The following steps are critical to achieving a more coordinated response to HIV:

1. Increase the coordination of HIV programs across the Federal government and between federal agencies and state, territorial, tribal, and local governments.

2. Develop improved mechanisms to monitor and report on progress toward achieving national goals.

Recommended Actions

Step 1: *Increase the coordination of HIV programs across the Federal Government and between Federal agencies and State, territorial, tribal, and local governments.*

Funding for HIV services is spread across multiple departments, including Health and Human Services (HHS), Housing and Urban Development (HUD), Justice, Veterans Affairs (VA), and Defense (Figure 5). Within HHS, in particular, responsibility for HIV programs is spread across multiple agencies including the Centers for Medicare & Medicaid Services (CMS), the Health Resources and Services Administration (HRSA), CDC, the Indian Health Service (IHS), the Food and Drug Administration, the Office of HIV/AIDS Policy, the Office of Minority Health, and others. Responsibility for HIV research is primarily carried by NIH, but CDC, VA, Department of Defense, and USAID also support research initiatives. This dispersion of responsibility is appropriate, as each agency has its own expertise, and different agencies operate different programs with varying purposes and with unique histories. Spreading the response to HIV across the Federal Government has helped our response to HIV. At the same time, it imposes costs and challenges us in getting the greatest results.

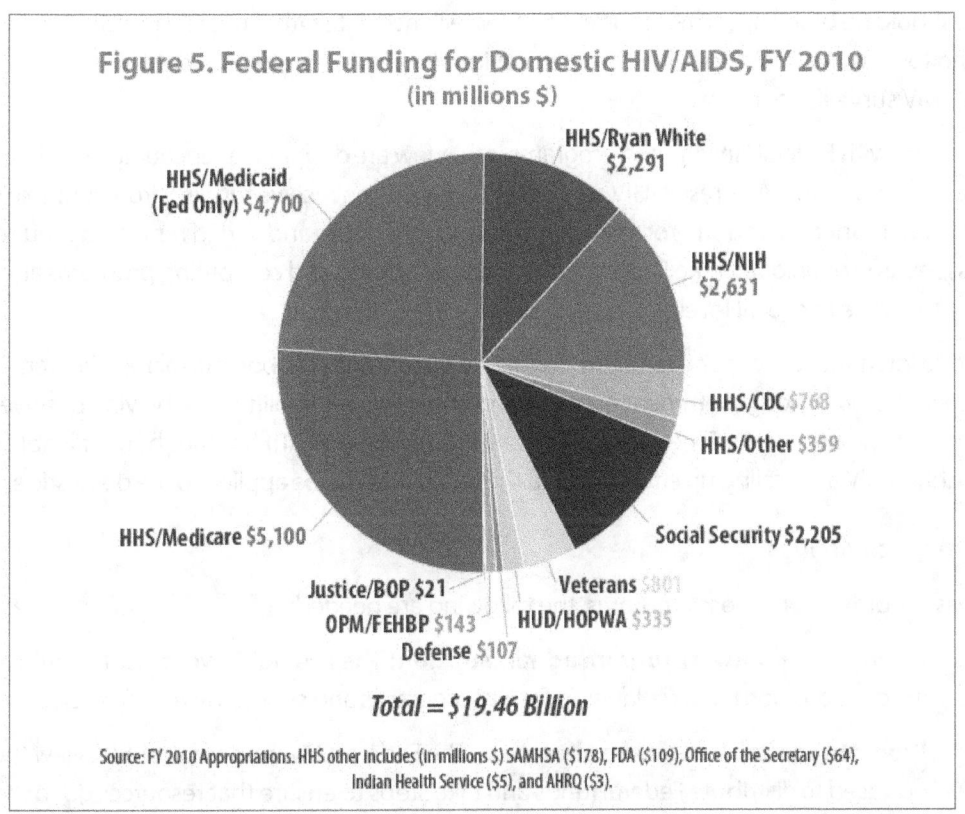

Figure 5. Federal Funding for Domestic HIV/AIDS, FY 2010
(in millions $)

HHS/Ryan White $2,291

HHS/Medicaid (Fed Only) $4,700

HHS/NIH $2,631

HHS/CDC $768

HHS/Other $359

HHS/Medicare $5,100

Social Security $2,205

Justice/BOP $21

Veterans $801

OPM/FEHBP $143

HUD/HOPWA $335

Defense $107

Total = $19.46 Billion

Source: FY 2010 Appropriations. HHS other includes (in millions $) SAMHSA ($178), FDA ($109), Office of the Secretary ($64), Indian Health Service ($5), and AHRQ ($3).

Roughly half of Federal funding for domestic HIV services flows through Medicaid and Medicare, two programs that are administered by the Centers for Medicare & Medicaid Services (CMS) (Figure 5). These programs provide essential guarantees of access to lifesaving medical care for all eligible beneficiaries, but the structure of the programs makes it difficult to adapt to HIV policy goals. Most services must be provided to all beneficiaries, and this limits the ability to target prevention and care services to high-risk populations. Moreover, data limitations make it hard to monitor people living with HIV as a distinct group. Other programs are more flexible, but competing rules, data collection requirements, and purposes create administrative burdens for the government, grantees and other external partners.

Laws governing HIV programs have changed over time, but have not all evolved in a way that places resources where they are most needed. For instance, some localities receive more funding for HIV prevention and care services than others despite having fewer persons living with HIV/AIDS. A recent analysis found that States with a low number of existing HIV/AIDS cases received the highest HIV prevention funding per case from CDC. The five States with 50 percent of the persons living with AIDS receive only 43 percent of CDC prevention funds for the Health Department Prevention, Expanded Testing Initiative, and Core Surveillance cooperative agreements, whereas the twenty jurisdictions that account for the last two percent of AIDS cases received nearly seven percent of the budget for these cooperative agreements.[160] If we are to target our efforts to more effectively address the epidemic, then resources to prevent HIV infection should be proportionate to disease burden. To achieve this, HIV prevention

_____

160. CDC analysis. Please refer to www.cdc.gov/hiv for the budget information and http://www.cdc.gov/hiv/topics/surveillance/resources/reports/ for surveillance data.

funding should be based upon more current HIV surveillance data rather than historical AIDS data. CDC is moving toward this goal and will be able to provide HIV in addition to AIDS data from all localities by the 2012 HIV surveillance report.

Another issue with Federal HIV funding programs is that few are designed to encourage efficient coordination across programs. As a result, HIV services providers often receive funding from multiple sources with different grant application processes and funding schedules, and varied reporting requirements. These issues are not unique at the Federal level, and overlapping and competing programs also hinder efforts at the State and local levels.

We need to integrate services and reduce redundancy, encourage collaboration across different levels of government and with nongovernment partners, and ensure accountability for achieving positive results. In this regard, the President's Emergency Plan for AIDS Relief (PEPFAR) has taught us valuable lessons about fighting HIV and scaling up efforts around the world that can be applied to the domestic epidemic.

Recommended Actions

To increase coordination across programs, the following are needed:

1.1 **Ensure coordinated program administration:** The Federal Government should increase its focus on coordinated planning for HIV programs and services across agencies.

1.2 **Promote equitable resource allocation:** The Federal Government should review the methods used to distribute Federal funds and take steps to ensure that resources go to the States and localities with the greatest need.

1.3 **Streamline and standardize data collection:** The Federal Government should take short and longer-term efforts to simplify grant administration activities, including work to standardize data collection, consolidating grant announcements, and grantee reporting requirements for Federal HIV programs.

Step 2: Develop improved mechanisms to monitor and report on progress toward achieving national goals.

The HIV epidemic in America requires a bold public health response. Annual AIDS deaths have declined, but the number of new infections has been static and the number of people living with HIV is growing. We need to be able to critically evaluate our current efforts to gauge the extent to which an impact is being made. Moreover, because of budget shortfalls at the state level, it is increasingly important that existing State and local efforts are concentrated and aligned with the Strategy goals. We need to measure the results of our efforts to reduce incidence and improve health outcomes to chart our progress in fighting HIV and AIDS nationally, and refine our response to this public health problem over time. This requires a monitoring system that evaluates the implementation of the Strategy, its progress, and the impact of the Strategy efforts. A system of regular public reporting will help to sustain public attention and support.

Recommended Actions

To monitor and communicate our progress, the following are needed:

2.1 **Provide rigorous evaluation of current programs and redirect resources to the most effective programs:** Prioritize programs that are 1) scientifically proven to reduce HIV infection, increase access to care, or reduce HIV-related disparities, 2) able to demonstrate sustained and long lasting (>1 year) outcomes toward achieving any of these goals, 3) scalable to produce desired outcomes at the community level, and 4) cost efficient.

2.2 **Provide regular public reporting:** Progress in reaching Strategy goals will be reported by the Federal Government through an annual report at the end of each year.

2.3 **Encourage States to provide regular progress reports:** The Federal Government will encourage States to provide annual reports to ONAP and HHS OS on progress made implementing their comprehensive HIV/AIDS plans. ONAP will incorporate the State reports into the national progress report at the end of each year.

Conclusion

HIV is a complex epidemic that creates many challenges and calls on all of us to take steps to protect ourselves, the communities where we live, and our Nation as a whole. There are many actions that should be taken, and there are many things that the United States has done well that offer lessons for future action. The development of a *National HIV/AIDS Strategy* is important because it is an effort to reflect on what is and is not working in order to increase the outcomes that we receive for our public and private investments. The Strategy is intended to refocus our existing efforts and deliver better results to the American people within current funding levels, as well as make the case for new investments. It is also a new attempt to set clear priorities and provide leadership for all public and private stakeholders to align their efforts toward a common purpose.

A perspective that arises out of the inclusive process used to develop this strategy leads us to recommend the following steps:

1. Resources will always be tight, and we will have to make tough choices about the most effective use of funds. Therefore, all resource allocation decisions for programs should be grounded in the latest epidemiological data about who is being most affected and other data that tell us which are the most urgent unmet needs to be addressed.

2. People living with HIV have unique experience that should be valued and relied upon as a critical source of input in setting policy.

3. Communities themselves are often the best equipped to make difficult trade-offs, and priority setting and resource allocation is best done as close to ground as possible.

4. Continued investment in research is needed. This includes biomedical research to develop new prevention strategies, safer, better therapies, and eventually a cure. There is also a need for additional health services research, operations research, and behavioral research and biomedical prevention research that have a population-level impact.

5. A commitment to innovation is needed to keep pace with an evolving epidemic, a scarcity of resources, and to support communities for which HIV is just one of many major challenges.

The steps outlined in this document merely provide a path forward. Because they are the result of broad-based engagement with Federal and community partners, we believe that they contain an informed wisdom from multiple perspectives and experiences. If they are to have any impact, individuals and groups all over the country will need to follow the path described and produce a more coordinated, collective response to HIV.

With government at all levels doing its part, a committed private sector, and leadership from people living with HIV and affected communities, the United States can dramatically reduce HIV transmission and better support people living with HIV and their families.